To be read

before being

Caregiver

in Nephrology

MARTIN STERLING

Table of contents

Chapter 7: Psychological support for nephrology patients   89

Chapter 8: Specific aspects of care for kidney transplant patients   101

Chapter 12: Technological innovation in nephrology   149

Chapter 13: Pediatrics in nephrology: specific care for children   163

Conclusion: The caregiver, a pillar of modern nephrology

« In the nephrology department, every gesture counts: caring for the patient's body also means calming his mind in the face of the complexity of kidney disease. »

Introduction

The importance of the nephrology caregiver

- **The key role of the caregiver in the care process**: Understanding the role of the caregiver in a multidisciplinary team.

The nursing auxiliary occupies a central position within the multidisciplinary nephrology team, providing a direct and continuous link between the patient, the other members of the nursing team, and all the healthcare professionals involved in the patient's care. Their role goes far beyond simply performing technical tasks, as they are the first to observe, listen and respond to the patient's immediate needs, often before the doctors or nurses intervene.

On a day-to-day basis, caregivers work closely with nurses, doctors, dieticians, physiotherapists and sometimes even psychologists. Each of these professionals brings a specific expertise, but the nursing auxiliary embodies the continuity of care. He is the one who ensures that the prescriptions and recommendations of these different players are applied when the patient needs them, thus guaranteeing consistency in care. They become the eyes and ears of the care team, being present at the patient's most intimate and vulnerable moments, whether for grooming, feeding or pain management.

The caregiver is often on the front line in detecting subtle changes in the patient's state of health, whether it's a variation in diuresis, an alteration in mood, or the appearance of clinical signs suggestive of a complication. This proximity enables him to alert nurses or doctors quickly, facilitating early and appropriate intervention. This fluid, permanent communication is one of the keys to success in a multidisciplinary team, as it avoids breaks in the care chain.

What's more, the nursing auxiliary plays a fundamental role in the human aspect of care, often where technicality and treatments take precedence. In a nephrology department, where patients are often confronted with heavy, repetitive treatments such as dialysis, they are a reassuring, soothing presence. They support patients in managing their day-to-day activities, but also in their emotional journey, supporting them in the face of the anguish associated with chronic illness, and providing an attentive ear. This relational dimension is indispensable, as it helps to maintain a crucial psychological balance in situations that can sometimes be trying for both the patient and his or her loved ones.

Finally, in a setting as complex as nephrology, the caregiver is also a key player in preventing complications. Whether it's ensuring rigorous hygiene to prevent infections in dialysis patients, or monitoring specific diets, the caregiver ensures that protocols are respected and dietary and therapeutic recommendations are implemented. In this way, they play an active role in the overall effectiveness of the care provided.

With their multi-faceted role, orderlies are the glue that holds together the harmony and efficiency of a multi-disciplinary nephrology team. His or her expertise, humanity and ability to work in synergy with all professionals make him or her an indispensable player in the holistic care of kidney patients.

- **Why choose nephrology?** Nephrology: The special features of this specialty and the challenges it presents.

Nephrology is a unique medical specialty in that it deals with kidney diseases, which affect an essential but often neglected organ in the public consciousness. The kidney plays a fundamental role in the body's equilibrium, eliminating waste products, regulating water and electrolytes, and managing the acid-base balance. When the kidneys fail to function properly, the consequences for the body are numerous and complex, affecting almost every system. This reality gives nephrology a demanding specificity: not only is it a medicine of regulation, but it requires a systemic approach, taking into account the whole organism and its interactions.

One of the first challenges facing nephrology is the diversity of the pathologies it covers. Renal diseases can be acute, such as acute renal failure, which occurs suddenly, or chronic, such as chronic renal failure, which progresses slowly but inexorably. What's more, they are often associated with other conditions such as high blood pressure, diabetes or cardiovascular disease, further complicating management. The caregiver, like the rest of the team, must not only understand these interactions, but also be able to identify the early signs of these complex pathologies, as renal failure often evolves insidiously, with discreet symptoms.

Another challenge is the heavy burden of treatment. Patients with chronic kidney failure are often faced with heavy treatments, such as dialysis, which is both life-saving and restrictive. Hemodialysis, for example, requires several sessions a week lasting several hours, with a heavy impact on patients' quality of life. Peritoneal dialysis, on the other hand, although carried out at home, requires rigorous personal care to avoid infections. Patients can feel exhausted by these repetitive treatments, and this is where the relational aspect of care becomes crucial. The caregiver, by virtue of his or her proximity to patients, must accompany them on this trying journey, not only physically, but also mentally. This support is essential to maintain morale and adherence to treatment, which is vital to the long-term management of kidney disease.

The management of kidney transplants is also a special area of nephrology, with its own challenges. While kidney transplantation is often perceived as an ideal "solution" for patients with end-stage renal failure, it is nonetheless a complex procedure, involving rigorous monitoring and heavy immunosuppressive treatments. Transplant patients must be closely monitored for any signs of rejection or infection, requiring constant vigilance on the part of the entire care team. The caregiver plays a key role in this daily monitoring, keeping an eye on the patient's general condition and promptly reporting any signs of deterioration.

What's more, nephrology is often a long-term specialty. Chronic kidney disease requires long-term follow-up, sometimes spanning decades, which creates a very special relationship between the patient and the healthcare team. This close relationship is both an asset and a challenge. For the caregiver, it's a question of maintaining constant attention and not falling into routine, despite the repetition of care. It also means knowing how to manage emotional fatigue, both for oneself and for the patient, in the face of the sometimes slow and inexorable progression of the disease. This psychological dimension is often just as important as managing the technical aspects of care, as depression and anxiety are frequent reactions in nephrology patients.

Finally, nephrology is a specialty that faces major inequalities. Chronic kidney disease is often linked to social factors, notably diabetes and hypertension, which are more prevalent in disadvantaged populations. This poses additional challenges in terms of prevention and therapeutic education, since it's not simply a question of providing treatment, but also of raising awareness and supporting patients who often lack the means or knowledge to adopt the necessary lifestyle changes. Caregivers play a fundamental role here, providing support and education to help patients better understand their illness and take charge of their own health.

- **Human and professional qualities required**: Empathy, rigor, patience and physical stamina.

The job of nephrology care assistant requires a set of human and professional qualities that go far beyond technical skills. These include empathy, rigor, patience and physical stamina, all of which are essential to meet the daily challenges of the department.

Empathy is perhaps the most fundamental quality in this specialty. Nephrology patients are often faced with serious chronic illnesses, which disrupt their daily lives and profoundly affect their state of mind. Whether the patient is on dialysis, awaiting a transplant or at the end of life, every interaction with the caregiver is tinged with vulnerability. Empathy enables the caregiver to connect with the patient, to understand their suffering beyond the visible symptoms, and to adapt care to their emotional needs. Sometimes, a simple gesture of reassurance or attentive listening can lighten the psychological load that the patient carries in silence. In a context as demanding as that of nephrology, where treatments are often long and results uncertain, empathy helps to humanize care and create a bond of trust that is essential to the quality of care.

However, this empathy cannot be effective without irreproachable professional rigor. Nephrology is a specialty where precise care is vital. Every task, however simple it may seem, must be carried out with the utmost attention. Whether it's taking vital signs, managing special diets, or monitoring a patient on dialysis, nothing can be left to chance. Rigor is also evident in the transmission of information to the care team. Because of their proximity to patients, orderlies are often the first to observe signs of complications, infections or deteriorating health. Neglected or poorly communicated observations can have serious consequences. Rigor thus becomes a form of collective responsibility, as it ensures that every member of the team has the necessary information to act at the right time and in the right way.

Patience, meanwhile, is an everyday virtue in this context. Nephrology patients, especially those suffering from chronic renal failure, often experience moments of intense frustration. The course of treatment is long, repetitive and sometimes discouraging. Dialysis sessions, strict dietary restrictions and chronic fatigue can be both morally and physically exhausting. Patients can be irritable, anxious or even resigned. At such times, the caregiver's patience is sorely tested. He must be able to respond calmly to tense situations, repeat the same explanations, and support the patient without allowing himself to be affected by the negative emotions that may emerge. Patience is not just about listening, but also about continuity of care. We have to accept that progress is often slow, and that remission, when possible, takes time.

Finally, physical stamina is an often underestimated but crucial aspect of a nephrology orderly's job. The job is physically demanding, involving long hours on your feet, a lot of moving around and regular physical exertion, such as mobilizing bedridden or frail patients. In a department where patients are often debilitated, it is necessary to frequently help them move around, whether it's to set them up for dialysis, mobilize them to prevent bedsores, or accompany them in their daily hygiene care. This repetition of physical effort, combined with the often staggered or extended working hours, requires good physical condition and great stamina. However, this physical stamina goes beyond mere strength. It's also a question of mental stamina, as the caregiver must be able to maintain his or her concentration and efficiency even during periods of intense fatigue or after trying days. This requires the ability to preserve oneself, manage one's energy and maintain a balance between professional and personal life.

Chapter 1

Nephrology in brief: Understanding the kidney and its functions

- **Anatomy and physiology of the kidney**: Basic concepts of glomerular filtration, reabsorption and tubular secretion. Glomerular filtration, reabsorption and tubular secretion are fundamental processes that enable the kidneys to maintain the body's internal equilibrium by managing waste elimination and regulating the volume and composition of body fluids. Understanding these mechanisms is essential to grasping the central role of the kidney in human physiology, and the consequences that kidney disease can have on the rest of the body.

Glomerular filtration: the first step in blood processing

The glomerular filtration process takes place in the glomeruli, tiny vascular structures located in the renal cortex. Each kidney contains around one million nephrons, the functional unit of the kidney, and each nephron begins with a glomerulus. The glomerulus consists of a network of capillaries enveloped by a structure called Bowman's capsule. The role of this structure is to filter the blood entering the kidneys via the renal arteries.

Under the effect of blood pressure, plasma containing water, electrolytes, small molecules (glucose, amino acids, etc.) and metabolic waste products, such as urea and creatinine, is pushed through the wall of the glomerular capillaries into Bowman's capsule. This filtered fluid, known as ultrafiltrate, resembles plasma, but without the large proteins and blood cells that are too bulky to pass through the filtration barrier. On average, the kidneys filter around 180 liters of blood per day, producing a large volume of ultrafiltrate, which is then modified in subsequent stages.

Tubular reabsorption: conserving what's essential

After glomerular filtration, the ultrafiltrate enters the renal tubule, where it undergoes complex modifications. The renal tubule is divided into several segments, each playing a specific role: the proximal convoluted tubule, the loop of Henle, the distal convoluted tubule, and finally, the collecting tube. Tubular reabsorption is a key process in this stage, as it recovers the useful substances that have been filtered by the glomerulus and returns them to the bloodstream. In fact, although 180 liters of liquid are filtered per day, only 1 to 2 liters of urine are excreted, which shows just how efficient reabsorption is.

In the proximal convoluted tubule, around 65% of filtered water and electrolytes (such as sodium and potassium) are reabsorbed, along with 100% of glucose and amino acids. This process is finely regulated by active and passive transport mechanisms, ensuring that only the necessary quantities are reabsorbed. For example, sodium pumps actively reabsorb sodium, while water is passively reabsorbed by osmosis. This segment of the tubule is also responsible for the reabsorption of bicarbonates, playing a crucial role in regulating the body's acid-base balance.

The loop of Henle then plays a specific role in urine concentration. In the descending part of the loop, water continues to be reabsorbed, while the ascending part is impermeable to water but actively reabsorbs sodium and chlorine. This mechanism creates an osmotic gradient which, in the more distal segments, allows even more water to be reabsorbed, especially under the influence of antidiuretic hormone (ADH), helping to maintain the body's water balance.

Tubular secretion: eliminating undesirable substances

While reabsorption recovers useful elements, tubular secretion actively removes undesirable substances that have not been efficiently filtered by the glomerulus. This process takes place mainly in the distal convoluted tubule and collecting tube. It involves ions such as potassium, hydrogen or ammonium, as well as metabolic waste products or drugs that must be excreted in the urine.

The secretion of protons (H+ ions) in the distal tubule plays a fundamental role in regulating the body's acid-base balance. By reabsorbing bicarbonate while secreting protons, the kidney helps maintain a stable blood pH. Moreover, potassium secretion is a crucial mechanism for avoiding hyperkalemia, a potentially dangerous condition that can affect cardiac activity.

A dynamic, regulated balance

The interaction between these three processes - glomerular filtration, tubular reabsorption and tubular secretion - enables the kidneys to finely regulate the composition of blood and body fluids. These mechanisms are influenced by factors such as blood pressure, blood volume, hormonal activity)such as aldosterone and ADH) and electrolyte concentration. When these processes function harmoniously, the body's water, electrolyte and acid-base balance is maintained.

However, when kidney function is impaired, as in chronic renal failure, these mechanisms become ineffective. The inability to filter blood properly leads to an accumulation of waste products and electrolyte imbalances, such as hyperkalemia or metabolic acidosis, which can rapidly become dangerous for the body.

- **Main kidney diseases**: renal failure, glomerular nephropathy, renal lithiasis.

Renal failure, glomerular nephropathy and renal lithiasis are three major categories of kidney disease, each with different mechanisms, symptoms and impact on the body, but all representing significant clinical challenges. These conditions affect the kidney in specific ways, compromising its ability to maintain the body's internal balance and ensure waste elimination. Understanding these pathologies enables us not only to grasp the complications they entail, but also to explore the care and treatment appropriate to each case.

Renal failure: progressive or sudden dysfunction

Renal failure, whether acute or chronic, represents a malfunction of the kidneys, preventing them from properly filtering blood and excreting metabolic waste products. This dysfunction may be progressive or occur suddenly.

Acute renal failure (ARF) is a sudden disorder in which the kidneys rapidly lose their ability to filter waste products and maintain fluid and electrolyte balance. It can be caused by a sudden drop in blood flow to the kidneys (as in hemodynamic shock), by renal toxicity due to drugs or toxins, or by urinary tract obstruction. In this type of failure, prompt intervention is crucial to avoid irreversible damage. Treatment focuses on correcting the underlying cause and supporting the kidneys during the critical phase.

Chronic renal failure (CRF), on the other hand, is a progressive and irreversible deterioration in kidney function, often due to diseases such as diabetes or hypertension. This process can extend over several years before symptoms become apparent, as the kidneys have a considerable capacity to adapt. However, once kidney function declines significantly, metabolic waste products such as urea and creatinine accumulate in the blood, causing symptoms such as fatigue, edema and electrolyte disorders. In advanced stages, CKD patients require dialysis or kidney

27

transplantation to replace lost kidney function. CKD treatment focuses on slowing the progression of the disease by controlling risk factors such as blood pressure and blood sugar levels.

Glomerular nephropathy: direct damage to renal filters

Glomerular nephropathies refer to a group of diseases affecting the glomeruli, the filtration units of the kidneys. These pathologies are often autoimmune or inflammatory, causing damage to glomerular structures and, consequently, poor blood filtration. As a result of this damage, proteins, blood or waste products can either be excreted in excess in the urine, or remain in the bloodstream, upsetting the body's internal balance.

Nephrotic syndrome is a frequent clinical manifestation of glomerular nephropathy. It is characterized by massive protein loss in the urine (proteinuria), leading to hypoproteinemia (low blood protein levels) and severe edema, particularly of the lower limbs and face. This loss of protein affects the osmotic balance and causes water retention in the tissues. This syndrome can be caused by autoimmune diseases such as lupus, or by specific conditions such as segmental and focal glomerulonephritis.

Nephritic syndrome, another type of glomerular nephropathy, is often the result of acute inflammation of the glomeruli. It manifests as hematuria (blood in the urine), hypertension, fluid retention and a moderate decline in renal function. This inflammation may be due to infection, autoimmune disease or post-infectious immunological reactions. In these cases, management aims to reduce inflammation, control associated symptoms, and prevent progression to chronic renal failure.

Although often difficult to diagnose, glomerular nephropathies represent a key field in nephrology because of their long-term implications for renal function. Their treatment often relies on immunosuppressants or corticosteroids to limit the inflammatory response and preserve glomerular function.

Kidney stones: painful but manageable

Renal lithiasis, commonly known as kidney stones, **are** hard mineral deposits that form in the kidneys from substances present in the urine, such as calcium, oxalate or uric acid. Kidney stones vary in size and composition, and when they migrate into the urinary tract, they can cause intense pain known as renal colic.

The formation of kidney stones **is** often favoured by high concentrations of certain substances in the urine, dehydration or metabolic abnormalities. Stones can obstruct the urinary tract, causing distension of the renal structures upstream of the obstruction and triggering severe pain. This pain may be accompanied by nausea, vomiting and, occasionally, haematuria. Depending on the size and location of the stone, treatment may vary. Small stones are often expelled naturally by the urinary flow, with good hydration and painkillers to relieve the pain. Larger stones, on the other hand, may require medical intervention, such as extracorporeal lithotripsy (which breaks the stone into smaller fragments using shock waves), or, in more serious cases, surgery.

Prevention of renal lithiasis relies mainly on abundant hydration to dilute mineral concentrations in the urine, as well as dietary adjustments, such as reducing sodium and oxalate intake, depending on the nature of the stone. Medication may also be prescribed to reduce the risk of recurrence, especially in people with a history of multiple stones.

- **The impact of kidney disease on the body**: hypertension, electrolyte imbalance, anemia.

Hypertension, electrolyte imbalances and anemia are three major complications that frequently accompany kidney disease, whether acute or chronic. Although seemingly distinct, these disorders are intimately linked to kidney function. When the kidneys no longer function properly, their ability to regulate blood pressure, balance electrolytes and stimulate red blood cell production is compromised. These three disorders represent crucial clinical challenges, as each can worsen renal failure and compromise other vital organs, notably the heart and circulatory system.

Hypertension: a vicious circle with kidney disease

High blood pressure (hypertension) is not only a major cause of kidney disease, but also one of its most common complications. The kidneys play a key role in regulating blood pressure by adjusting the volume of fluid in the body and releasing hormones, such as renin, which influence the constriction of blood vessels. When kidney function is impaired, this delicate balance is disturbed, and blood pressure can rise uncontrollably.

Hypertension itself can cause progressive damage to the blood vessels in the kidneys, a phenomenon known as nephroangiosclerosis, which further worsens kidney function. It's a vicious circle: kidney disease leads to hypertension, and hypertension accelerates kidney deterioration. As the kidneys lose their ability to filter blood efficiently, water and salt retention increases, leading to increased blood volume and additional pressure on artery walls. This makes hypertension a difficult complication to manage, often requiring multiple medications to control.

Patients suffering from chronic renal failure need to be closely monitored to avoid excessive elevation of blood pressure, which could damage not only the kidneys, but also the heart, increasing the risk of stroke or heart failure. Treatment of hypertension in nephrology often relies on a combination of diuretics, which reduce fluid volume, and inhibitors of the renin-angiotensin system, which reduce pressure in the renal glomeruli.

Electrolyte imbalance: a threat to homeostasis

The kidneys play a central role in the regulation of electrolytes, such as sodium, potassium, calcium and phosphorus, which are essential for water balance, nerve and muscle function, and many metabolic processes. When the kidneys are damaged, their ability to maintain this balance is compromised, leading to electrolyte imbalances that can have serious consequences for the body.

Hyperkalemia, or increased potassium levels in the blood, is one of the most worrying electrolyte imbalances in patients with kidney disease. Potassium is normally excreted by the kidneys, but in renal failure this excretion is diminished, leading to a progressive accumulation of potassium in the blood. Hyperkalemia is particularly dangerous, as it can lead to life-threatening cardiac arrhythmias. For this reason, patients with renal failure should follow potassium-restricted diets, avoid certain drugs (such as non-steroidal anti-inflammatory drugs), and be monitored regularly by blood tests.

Hypocalcemia, or low calcium levels, and hyperphosphatemia, or excess phosphorus, are also common in patients with chronic kidney disease. This is due to the kidneys' inability to activate vitamin D, which is necessary for calcium absorption in the intestine, and to excrete phosphorus correctly. These imbalances can affect bone metabolism, leading to renal osteodystrophy, which weakens bones and increases the risk of fractures. Treatments for these imbalances include calcium supplements, phosphorus binders and active forms of vitamin D to restore mineral balance and prevent long-term complications.

Anemia: a silent but debilitating consequence

Anemia is a frequent complication of renal failure, particularly in the advanced stages. In addition to their role in filtering waste products and regulating electrolytes, the kidneys are also responsible for producing erythropoietin (EPO), a hormone that stimulates the production of red blood cells in the bone marrow. As kidney function declines, EPO production decreases, leading to a drop in the number of red blood cells in the blood and, consequently, a reduction in the blood's ability to transport oxygen to tissues.

Anemia in patients with chronic renal failure often manifests itself as intense fatigue, shortness of breath, dizziness and reduced ability to perform daily activities. It also contributes to the worsening of cardiovascular disease, forcing the heart to work harder to compensate for the lack of oxygen, which can lead to cardiac hypertrophy and increase the risk of heart failure.

Treatment of renal anemia relies primarily on the administration of erythropoiesis-stimulating agents (ESAs), which replace the function of EPO, as well as iron supplements, as iron deficiency can exacerbate anemia in these patients. It's also essential to monitor hemoglobin levels regularly to adjust treatment, as correcting anemia too quickly or excessively can also have adverse effects.

A delicate balance: interdependence of complications

These three complications - hypertension, electrolyte imbalances and anemia - are not isolated phenomena. They interact with each other, often exacerbating each other's negative effects. For example, hypertension exacerbates renal failure, intensifying electrolyte imbalances, while anemia and hyperkalemia increase the cardiac risks associated with hypertension. These interconnections make the management of kidney disease a complex exercise in constant rebalancing.

Chapter 2

The daily life of a nephrology ward orderly

- **First steps in the department**: familiarize yourself with the department's organization and specific features.

Familiarizing yourself with the organization and specifics of a nephrology department is a crucial step for any newcomer, whether an orderly or any other member of the nursing staff. The nephrology department has unique features due to the specific needs of patients with chronic or acute kidney disease, as well as the highly technical and rigorous nature of care. Understanding the organization of the department and its specific features will enable you not only to integrate quickly, but also to contribute effectively to optimal patient care, while respecting protocols and working in synergy with the multidisciplinary team.

An organization structured around comprehensive renal patient care

The nephrology department is often organized into several units or sectors, each responding to specific patient needs. Typically, there is an inpatient unit for acute renal failure or severe complications, a dedicated dialysis sector (hemodialysis and peritoneal dialysis), and an outpatient sector for regular consultations and management of patients with chronic kidney disease. Each sector operates in an interconnected fashion, as patients may need to move from one unit to another during the course of their treatment, depending on the evolution of their state of health.

One of the major specificities of this department is the repetitive nature of care for certain patients, particularly those undergoing dialysis. Hemodialysis sessions, for example, take place several times a week and last several hours. This regularity of care implies a well-honed organization, with fixed time slots, strict protocols for the preparation of dialysis equipment, and continuous monitoring of patients during treatment. Familiarity with this routine is essential for the caregiver, as each step must be meticulously respected to ensure that sessions run smoothly and avoid complications.

Coordinated, multidisciplinary care

One of the most striking features of the nephrology department is the importance of multidisciplinary teamwork. The care of kidney patients is not limited to the management of their failing kidneys, but encompasses a global vision of their health. Nursing assistants, nurses, nephrologists, dieticians, psychologists, physiotherapists and other healthcare professionals work closely together to provide comprehensive care that takes into account the many co-morbidities associated with kidney disease.

The nursing auxiliary plays a key role in this organization, as the hub of daily care. They are often the first to observe patients and report subtle changes in their state of health. To do this, they must not only be attentive, but also master the particularities of renal care, such as monitoring diuresis, keeping track of vitals (blood pressure, weight, fluid balance), and preventing infections, especially in patients with catheters or arteriovenous fistulas.

The importance of vigilance and precision

The nephrology department demands constant vigilance and rigorous attention to detail. Patients undergoing dialysis, for example, are often at high risk of complications, such as hypotension, cramps, or infections linked to vascular access devices. To minimize these risks, every procedure must be precise and every parameter carefully controlled. This means knowing the protocols in force, understanding alarms and warning signs, and knowing how to react quickly in the event of a problem.

Handling medical devices, such as catheters or dialysis machines, is an integral part of nephrology work. Nurses must be trained in the use and management of this specific equipment, particularly with regard to sterilization, fistula maintenance and the prevention of nosocomial infections. Strict adherence to hygiene procedures is vital, as dialysis patients are often immunocompromised and particularly vulnerable to infection.

Patient support and therapeutic education

Another fundamental aspect of the organization of the nephrology department is the long-term care of patients, particularly those suffering from chronic renal failure. These patients are often hospitalized on a regular basis, or come frequently for their dialysis sessions. Kidney disease imposes major lifestyle changes, and the caregiver plays an essential role in patients' therapeutic education.

It's not just a question of providing technical care, but also of helping patients understand their illness and treatment. For example, the caregiver can explain the importance of following dietary recommendations (in particular to limit salt, potassium or phosphorus intake) or water restrictions, and of recognizing the warning signs of complications. By providing this educational dimension, the caregiver helps to empower the patient, reinforcing adherence to treatment and improving long-term quality of life.

Emotional and relational management

Last but not least, relational and emotional aspects play a vital role in the organization of the department. Nephrology patients, especially those undergoing dialysis, often experience periods of discouragement, anxiety and frustration in the face of difficult treatments and uncertainties about their state of health. The nephrology department is therefore a place where caregivers need to demonstrate great empathy and constant support.

By working closely with patients on a daily basis, caregivers often become a reassuring point of reference for them. They play an active role in creating an environment of trust and benevolence, which is essential in helping patients overcome difficult moments and accept their therapeutic journey. This emotional support is an essential aspect of nephrology care, as it directly influences patients' well-being and their ability to live with their illness.

- **Welcoming and seating the patient**: the importance of physical and psychological comfort.

The physical and psychological comfort of patients is an essential dimension of care, particularly in a department as demanding as nephrology. Patients suffering from kidney disease, whether chronic renal failure, glomerulonephritis or other renal conditions, are confronted with long, repetitive and sometimes invasive treatments, which can profoundly affect their physical and mental well-being. In this context, the importance of comfort, both physical and psychological, cannot be underestimated, as it plays a crucial role in patients' quality of life and adherence to care.

Physical comfort: relieving suffering and preventing complications

Physical comfort is one of the first aspects to be taken into account when caring for nephrology patients. These patients, particularly those on dialysis, spend long hours immobile, often several times a week, connected to a machine that temporarily replaces the function of their kidneys. This prolonged immobility can lead to muscular pain, discomfort in the back, arms or legs, and intense fatigue. For a caregiver, ensuring a patient's physical comfort begins with simple but essential gestures, such as ensuring that the patient is correctly positioned in bed or in a chair, adjusting pillows and limb support, and suggesting solutions to relieve muscular tension.

In nephrology, physical comfort is not limited to the postural aspect. It also includes pain management, which can be a recurring problem for these patients. Muscle cramps, for example, are common in dialysis patients due to electrolyte imbalances induced by extracorporeal filtration. The caregiver needs to be alert to these manifestations and react quickly by adjusting the patient's position or applying relieving measures such as massage or warm compresses. Similarly, attention to the skin, particularly in bedridden or dialysis patients, is essential to prevent bedsores and skin irritation, complications which can seriously compromise physical well-being.

Regular monitoring of medical devices also contributes to this comfort. For example, patients with arteriovenous fistulas, essential for haemodialysis, require careful care to prevent infection or thrombosis. A poorly maintained catheter can cause pain and severe complications, directly affecting patient comfort. Vigilance and rigorous maintenance of vascular access points are integral to maintaining optimal physical comfort.

Psychological comfort: soothing anxiety and boosting morale

Patients' psychological comfort is just as important, if not more so, than their physical comfort. Living with a chronic kidney disease, undergoing heavy and repetitive treatments such as dialysis, or waiting for a kidney transplant, are situations that generate great anxiety, uncertainty and sometimes discouragement. Psychological stress can be exacerbated when patients feel isolated or misunderstood in their suffering. This is where the caregiver's human and empathetic support plays a crucial role.

Psychological comfort starts with a reassuring presence. Simply listening to the patient's concerns, answering their questions or calmly explaining the stages of care can go a long way to alleviating anxiety. In nephrology, where patients are often subjected to strict diets, fluid restrictions or repetitive care sessions, the caregiver's role is also to remind patients of their therapeutic objectives, encourage them to maintain their efforts and highlight the small victories they achieve on a daily basis.

This constant accompaniment helps to create an environment of trust in which the patient feels supported.

Familiarity with the patient also plays a fundamental role in maintaining psychological comfort. In nephrology, where patients return regularly for their care, a human bond is forged with the nursing staff. This relationship of trust, based on empathy and understanding of individual needs, enables patients to feel recognized, listened to and cared for in a personalized way. This is particularly true for chronic patients, who have to live with their illness over the long term. Knowing that they can count on attentive, caring caregivers enables them to accept their condition better, and to approach their care with less apprehension.

Finally, psychological comfort means taking into account the emotional dimension of kidney disease. Patients can sometimes experience the frustration of seeing their state of health deteriorate despite treatment, or the anguish of waiting for a transplant that is long in coming. Some may also develop a sense of loss of autonomy, or even dependence, which can affect their morale. The caregiver, through his or her regular presence and psychological support, can help overcome these difficult moments by offering active listening and emotional support. Sometimes, it's simply a matter of creating a space in which patients can express their fears or doubts, without judgment, but with empathy.

The interplay between physical and psychological comfort

Physical and psychological comfort are inseparable and mutually reinforcing. A patient who feels well physically will be better able to cope with the psychological challenges associated with his or her illness. Conversely, a patient whose worries and anxieties are alleviated will be better able to cope with the physical discomforts associated with his or her treatment. Care must therefore be considered holistically, taking into account the interdependence of these two dimensions.

In this context, the caregiver plays a fundamental role by adopting a benevolent, holistic approach to care. For example, providing a calm and soothing environment, adjusting light or room temperature, ensuring that the patient has pleasant distractions during the dialysis session (such as a book, music, or the chance to talk to someone), all contribute to improving psychological comfort while meeting immediate physical needs.

- **Collaborate with the multidisciplinary team**: work in synergy with nurses, nephrologists, dieticians and physiotherapists.

Working in synergy with nurses, nephrologists, dieticians and physiotherapists is essential to ensure comprehensive, coherent patient care in the nephrology department. The nature of kidney disease and its many complications calls for a multidisciplinary approach, with each healthcare professional bringing his or her own specific expertise to bear. However, the effectiveness of this collaboration depends not only on complementary skills, but above all on communication and coordination between the various members of the healthcare team.

The caregiver's key role in care synergy

The nursing auxiliary occupies a central position in this teamwork. Their constant proximity to patients makes them the first observers of their condition on a daily basis. They are often the first to detect subtle changes in their physical or psychological state, whether signs of fatigue, anxiety, pain or complications such as edema or variations in blood pressure. These observations are crucial and need to be communicated promptly to nurses, nephrologists and other team members, so that they can adjust treatment or care accordingly.

The caregiver's role is not limited to monitoring patients. They are also responsible for a wide range of basic care tasks, such as grooming, settling the patient, and managing vital signs (blood pressure, weight, diuresis). Every action taken and every piece of data collected is of vital importance to the patient's progress, and must be shared with the nursing team. This information is passed on both orally when the teams take over, and through notes in the patient's medical file. The clarity and precision of this information is essential to enable the team to work smoothly and make informed decisions.

Close collaboration with nurses

The collaboration between nursing assistants and nurses is particularly close. These two professionals work side by side to ensure the day-to-day care of patients. While the nurse focuses on technical and medical care, such as medication management, monitoring infusions or vascular access for dialysis, the orderly is often responsible for the more practical and relational aspect of care.

However, this distinction of roles must not create barriers. Caregivers and nurses must constantly exchange information to ensure consistent, comprehensive care. For example, the caregiver may alert the nurse to early signs of complications (such as hypotension during a dialysis session), or inform the nurse that the patient has expressed pain or discomfort. In return, the nurse can guide the caregiver on adjustments to be made in daily care, particularly in terms of special monitoring or specific precautions to be taken.

Interaction with nephrologists: an essential link

The nephrologist is the specialist physician who oversees the patient's overall treatment. His role is to assess the progression of kidney disease, prescribe treatments, and decide on any necessary adjustments. Although the caregiver is not directly involved in medical decisions, his or her role as observer is crucial in providing the nephrologist with valuable information on the patient's condition. For example, if a patient shows signs of fluid imbalance (such as edema or decreased diuresis), or complains of abnormal fatigue, these may signal worsening renal failure or a need to adjust dialysis.

By working in close collaboration with nephrologists, caregivers play an indirect role in optimizing treatments. During medical visits or team meetings, the caregiver's observations are taken into account to fine-tune therapeutic decisions. This cooperation is based on mutual trust and recognition of the key role each professional plays in patient care.

The contribution of dieticians: a partnership for nutrition

Nutrition plays a central role in the management of kidney disease, as patients often have to follow strict diets to control their salt, potassium, phosphorus and protein intake. The dietician, in collaboration with the nephrologist, is responsible for designing nutritional plans tailored to the specific needs of each patient. However, if these recommendations are to be applied effectively, close cooperation with the caregiver is essential.

The caregiver is in the front line of ensuring that patients comply with dietary restrictions. Not only do they have to monitor dietary intakes, but they must often explain and remind patients of the reasons for these restrictions. For example, in a dialysis patient, excess potassium can lead to serious complications, such as heart problems. The caregiver must therefore be vigilant in pointing out any deviations or difficulties the patient may encounter in following his or her diet. In return, the dietician can adjust the recommendations based on the caregiver's observations of the patient's appetite or nutritional status.

Cooperation with physiotherapists: optimizing patient mobility

Patients with kidney disease, especially those on dialysis, often suffer from chronic fatigue, loss of mobility, and muscular degradation due to inactivity or nutritional imbalances. The role of the physiotherapist is therefore essential in helping these patients maintain their physical strength and mobility, and prevent complications associated with immobility, such as bedsores or venous thrombosis.

The caregiver works in synergy with the physiotherapist to encourage patients to perform simple mobilization exercises, whether in bed, in a chair or walking. In some cases, the caregiver directly assists the physiotherapist during rehabilitation sessions. Between visits from the physiotherapist, they also ensure continuity of care by helping patients with their daily exercises, mobilizing them regularly, or ensuring that they change position to avoid complications associated with prolonged bed rest. This cooperation ensures better physical recovery and an improvement in patients' overall well-being.

Chapter 3

Basic care for nephrology patients

- **Patient grooming and hygiene**: managing fragile skin and preventing pressure sores.

Managing fragile skin and preventing pressure sores are crucial elements of patient care, particularly in the nephrology department, where many patients are bedridden, dialyzed or have reduced mobility. These situations considerably increase the risk of skin complications such as pressure sores, which not only cause intense pain, but can also lead to serious infections and affect the patient's general condition. For a caregiver, careful monitoring of the skin and the implementation of appropriate prevention strategies are essential to protect skin integrity and improve patients' quality of life.

Understanding skin fragility in nephrology patients

Patients with chronic kidney disease, particularly those on dialysis, often have more fragile skin due to multiple factors. The accumulation of toxins in the blood, due to reduced kidney function, can alter the structure and function of the skin, making it drier, thinner and more prone to irritation. In addition, frequent electrolyte imbalances, as well as the water restrictions imposed on these patients, often lead to skin dehydration, making it more vulnerable to damage.

Skin fragility is accentuated by prolonged bed rest, particularly in patients with advanced kidney disease or those who have undergone major surgery. Immobility, combined with the constant pressure exerted on certain areas of the body, notably the heels, buttocks and elbows, increases the risk of pressure ulcer formation. These sores develop when blood circulation is compromised in an area of prolonged pressure, leading to tissue necrosis.

The importance of pressure sore prevention

The prevention of pressure sores is a major issue in the care of frail patients. Once formed, these wounds can be difficult to treat, especially in dialysis patients, who often have difficulty healing due to toxin accumulation, malnutrition or circulatory disorders. Preventing pressure sores is therefore not only a priority to preserve patient comfort and health, but also to avoid serious complications, such as infections that can spread rapidly.

Prevention strategies: regular mobilization

One of the most effective ways of preventing pressure sores is to reduce the pressure exerted on at-risk areas by regularly mobilizing patients. Patients who are bedridden or have reduced mobility should be changed position at least every two hours to prevent pressure points from forming. This task often falls to the caregiver, who is responsible for regularly repositioning the patient, while ensuring that movements are gentle enough not to cause skin micro-lesions.

Mobilization doesn't just mean changing the patient's position in bed. It may also involve helping them to get up and walk, if this is possible, or moving them into a wheelchair. This type of active mobilization, when feasible, stimulates blood circulation and strengthens muscle resistance, reducing the risk of pressure sores while improving the patient's general condition. For patients who can't move around on their own, the caregiver must use adapted techniques, sometimes in collaboration with physiotherapists, to avoid creating overly prolonged pressure points.

Use of preventive devices: anti-bedsore mattresses and cushions

In addition to position changes, the use of suitable devices, such as dynamic air mattresses or anti-bedsore cushions, is essential to reduce pressure on at-risk areas. These devices distribute the body's weight more evenly and relieve the most exposed pressure points. Air mattresses, for example, alternate pressure zones through cycles of inflation and deflation, helping to maintain adequate blood circulation in skin tissue.

The caregiver is often responsible for checking the condition of these devices, adjusting them if necessary, and ensuring that they are used correctly. They may also recommend the use of additional cushions or supports, such as heel cushions or elbow pads, to protect particularly sensitive areas in some patients.

Skin care: moisturizing and careful observation

Another key aspect of pressure sore prevention is daily skin care. In nephrology patients, the skin tends to be dry and dehydrated, making it more vulnerable to irritation and cracking. It is therefore crucial to apply moisturizers or emollients regularly to keep the skin supple. This care should be carried out gently, avoiding excessive rubbing, especially in high-risk areas.

Hygiene is also a fundamental factor in pressure sore prevention. Caregivers must ensure that the skin is clean and dry, particularly after washing or in the event of incontinence. Prolonged dampness can weaken the skin barrier and encourage maceration, thus increasing the risk of pressure sores. Products used for cleansing should be gentle and suitable for fragile skin, to avoid further irritation.

Careful observation of the skin is also an integral part of the caregiver's role. It is essential to regularly examine at-risk areas such as the heels, buttocks, hips and elbows, in order to detect the first signs of pressure sores. Persistent redness, an area that is warm or cold to the touch, or the beginnings of a skin lesion are all warning signs that should be reported immediately to the nurse or doctor. Early intervention is often the key to preventing these signs from developing into deeper, more difficult-to-treat ulcers.

A global approach to care

Pressure sore prevention is not limited to technical gestures or the use of specific equipment. It is part of an overall approach to care, which takes into account the patient's physical and psychological well-being. For a patient to be effectively protected against pressure sores, it is essential that they are well nourished, well hydrated and that their general condition is carefully managed. The caregiver plays a crucial role in this holistic approach, looking after not only the patient's skin, but also his or her comfort, mobility, nutrition and morale.

- **Mobility support and prevention of loss of autonomy**: Mobilization techniques and adapted exercises.

Mobilization techniques and adapted exercises play a central role in the management of patients with kidney disease, particularly those who are bedridden, on dialysis or suffering from mobility limitations. Regular mobilization and exercise are essential to prevent a wide range of complications, such as pressure sores, deep vein thrombosis, loss of muscle mass and respiratory disorders. In nephrology, where patients often face long and demanding treatments such as dialysis, maintaining a certain level of physical activity is not only beneficial for the body, but also for psychological well-being.

The importance of mobilization for nephrology patients

Patients suffering from kidney failure, whether on hemodialysis or in the advanced stages of the disease, can often feel exhausted, weakened and gradually lose their mobility. This loss of mobility may be due to chronic fatigue, disease-induced muscle weakness, or prolonged periods of bed rest. However, inactivity is a vicious circle: the longer a patient remains immobile, the more his or her physical condition deteriorates, making recovery even more difficult. Mobilization and adapted physical exercise are therefore essential to counteract this effect, maintain muscle strength and promote blood circulation.

For a caregiver, mobilizing patients is a crucial daily task. It involves more than simply moving or repositioning patients in bed, but also encouraging them to participate actively, according to their abilities. The aim is to maintain the highest possible level of autonomy, while ensuring patient safety and comfort.

Passive and active mobilization techniques

Mobilization techniques fall into two main categories: passive mobilization, where the caregiver directly helps the patient to move, and active mobilization, where the patient is encouraged to perform movements on his or her own.

Passive mobilization is often used for patients who are totally or partially unable to move on their own, such as those who are bedridden or suffering from severe pain. In these cases, the caregiver performs gentle, controlled movements on the patient's limbs to prevent joint stiffness, maintain muscle flexibility, and stimulate blood circulation. This may include flexion and extension of the arms and legs, gentle rotation of the ankles, elbows or wrists, and exercises to soften the hips and shoulders. These simple gestures are essential to prevent muscle contractures and preserve joint mobility, even in patients who are unable to stand up.

With **active mobilization**, patients are encouraged to perform their own movements, with or without the assistance of a caregiver. For some patients, this may involve simple movements such as raising and lowering the arms or bending the knees while sitting or lying down. For others, who are more mobile, it may include gentle muscle-strengthening exercises, stretching movements, or even short walks in the hallway. The aim of active mobilization is to stimulate muscular activity, improve blood circulation and preserve cardiorespiratory function as far as possible.

Adapted exercises: maintaining strength and flexibility

Exercises suitable for nephrology patients vary according to their state of health, level of fatigue and capacity for movement. However, there are simple exercises that can be performed in bed or in a seated position, even by weakened patients. These exercises are often carried out in collaboration with a physiotherapist, but the caregiver plays a key role in ensuring continuity and regularity of exercise sessions.

Muscle-strengthening exercises are important for maintaining muscle mass, particularly in dialysis patients, who are often subject to progressive muscle wasting. These exercises can include flexion-extension movements of the legs and arms, leg lifts while lying down, or the use of elastic bands to add gentle resistance to the movements. These exercises help preserve muscle strength, which is crucial for patients' independence in daily activities such as getting out of bed or walking.

Breathing exercises are also important for bedridden patients or those with reduced respiratory capacity. Deep breathing exercises, such as slow inhalation followed by prolonged exhalation, help to improve lung function, prevent respiratory infections, and oxygenate the blood more effectively. Encouraging patients to practice regular breathing exercises is essential, especially after a period of prolonged immobilization.

Gentle stretching exercises keep muscles and joints supple. These movements help avoid muscle stiffness and prevent joint pain, which often occurs after periods of inactivity. They can include arm and leg stretches, gentle wrist and ankle rotations, and back and shoulder stretches to release accumulated tension.

The importance of autonomy and motivation

For nephrology patients, maintaining some form of autonomy is essential, not only physically, but also psychologically. Appropriate exercise and regular mobilization help patients to maintain their ability to perform simple actions, such as getting up or moving around, giving them a sense of control over their bodies and their state of health. Encouraging patients to take an active part in their rehabilitation is one way of motivating them to stay involved in their own care.

The caregiver plays a key role in this dynamic. It's not just a question of physically guiding patients, but also of encouraging them, reassuring them and giving them confidence in their abilities. Some patients, especially those suffering from anxiety or depression linked to their illness, may be reluctant to move or make any effort. In such cases, it's important to understand their reluctance and suggest simple, accessible **exercises**, while emphasizing the long-term benefits of physical activity.

Safety first: risk-free support

Mobilization and physical exercises should always be performed with the patient's abilities and limitations in mind. It is essential to proceed gently and carefully, ensuring that the patient feels neither pain nor discomfort. The caregiver must ensure that movements are carried out correctly, avoid any over-exertion that could lead to a fall or injury, and be alert to any signs of fatigue or discomfort in the patient.

When patients are mobilized to stand or walk, the caregiver must ensure that the environment is safe: the floor must be clear, the patient must be properly supported, and, if necessary, devices such as walkers or wheelchairs must be used to ensure the patient's stability.

- **Monitoring of vitals**: Blood pressure measurement, diuresis measurement, water balance management.

Taking blood pressure, measuring diuresis and managing fluid balance are three essential tasks in the daily monitoring of nephrology patients. These parameters are intimately linked to renal health and the kidneys' ability to regulate fluids and blood pressure in the body. Careful and rigorous monitoring of these elements not only enables us to monitor the progression of kidney disease, but also to prevent and detect serious complications, such as hypertension, edema or dehydration, at an early stage. As a caregiver, being trained and vigilant in managing these aspects is crucial to patient safety and well-being.

Blood pressure: a key indicator in nephrology

In nephrology, blood pressure measurement is an essential daily routine, as hypertension is one of the main causes and consequences of kidney disease. The kidneys play a central role in regulating blood pressure, and kidney dysfunction can lead to disturbances in this system. High blood pressure can accelerate the progression of kidney failure, while low blood pressure, particularly during dialysis, can lead to malaise and serious complications.

When taking blood pressure readings, caregivers must ensure that they are carried out under optimum conditions to obtain reliable readings. The patient should be in a sitting or lying position, at rest for several minutes, and the arm used for measurement should be supported at heart level. Using the right cuff size is also essential to avoid measurement errors. Each measurement must be accurately recorded in the patient's file, as it will be used to adjust treatments and assess overall health.

In dialysis, blood pressure monitoring is particularly critical before, during and after the session. During dialysis, a rapid drop in blood pressure can occur, due to the loss of blood volume associated with the removal of excess fluids. This can lead to symptoms such as dizziness, nausea or weakness, and requires prompt intervention by the care team. Monitoring blood pressure at regular intervals is essential to prevent these complications and adjust the dialysis session accordingly.

Measuring diuresis: assessing renal function

Measuring diuresis, i.e. the volume of urine produced by the patient over a given period of time, is a direct indicator of renal function. Healthy kidneys produce a quantity of urine adapted to the body's water intake and condition, but in patients suffering from kidney disease, this capacity is often impaired. Insufficient diuresis (oliguria) or a total absence of urine production (anuria) are signs of deteriorating renal function, while excessive urine production (polyuria) may indicate poor fluid reabsorption by the kidneys.

In practice, diuresis is measured by collecting the patient's urine over a 24-hour period, or over a shorter period in specific contexts, such as post-dialysis monitoring. This task is often delegated to the caregiver, who ensures that the collection is carried out rigorously. The patient must be informed of the importance of retaining all the urine produced, and of not omitting to collect even small quantities. Once the urine has been collected, the total volume is accurately measured and recorded in the medical record.

This measurement is not only an indicator of the kidneys' ability to filter blood. It can also be used to assess the efficacy of treatments, particularly in patients on diuretics, and to monitor patient response after dialysis or medical treatment. Diuresis is also a critical indicator for adjusting fluid intake, as it determines the patient's ability to eliminate excess water.

Managing the water balance: an essential balance

Water balance management involves balancing the patient's water intake and loss. This balance is crucial in patients with kidney disease, as their kidneys are no longer able to regulate body fluids effectively. Excess water in the body can cause edema, hypertension and aggravate cardiac complications, while dehydration can lead to hypotension, general weakness and severe electrolyte imbalances.

The water balance is calculated by comparing water intake (liquids ingested by the patient, including drinks, but also water contained in food) with losses (urine, sweat, respiration, etc.). In nephrology, monitoring this balance is particularly rigorous, especially for patients on dialysis. Indeed, these patients often have to limit their fluid intake to avoid water overload, as their kidneys can no longer eliminate excess water efficiently.

The nursing auxiliary plays a fundamental role in this management. First and foremost, he or she must ensure accurate recording of all the patient's fluid intake. This includes not only water and beverages, but also water-rich foods such as soups and fruit. Secondly, he must monitor losses, particularly diuresis, but also, in some cases, losses through vomiting or diarrhea.

For patients on dialysis, water balance is also managed during treatment sessions, when some of the excess fluid is removed by the dialysis machine. Before each session, the patient's weight is measured to estimate the amount of fluid to be removed. The aim is to achieve a so-called "dry weight", corresponding to a state where the patient has neither excess fluid nor dehydration. Monitoring weight before and after dialysis is therefore another of the caregiver's responsibilities, helping to assess the patient's water balance.

Constant vigilance: detecting signs of imbalance

Monitoring blood pressure, diuresis and fluid balance is not just a technical task; it also requires constant vigilance on the part of the caregiver, who must be able to interpret the signs of imbalance. Blood pressure that is too high or too low, a sudden drop in diuresis, or rapid weight gain between two dialysis sessions may indicate a deterioration in the patient's condition, and must be reported immediately to the nurse or doctor.

Signs of fluid imbalance, such as edema, shortness of breath, unusual fatigue or dry mouth, should also be carefully monitored, as they may be early signs of fluid overload or dehydration. Working closely with the nursing team, the caregiver helps to prevent serious complications and adjust treatments to maintain the patient's fluid balance and stability.

Chapter 4

Clinical monitoring in nephrology

- **Warning signs to watch out for**: edema, hypotension, anuria, hyperkalemia.

Edema, hypotension, anuria and hyperkalemia are frequent clinical manifestations in patients with kidney disease, whether acute or chronic renal failure. These symptoms are often interconnected, stemming directly from the dysfunction of the kidneys, which can no longer effectively regulate body fluids, blood pressure and electrolytes. Each symptom represents an important warning sign that the body's water and electrolyte balance has been compromised. For a caregiver, being able to recognize and understand these manifestations is essential, as they can develop rapidly and have serious consequences for the patient's health.

Edema: the accumulation of fluid in tissues

Edema is a visible swelling of tissues, usually in the lower limbs, ankles, face or abdomen. They result from excessive fluid accumulation in the interstitial spaces, i.e. between cells. This water retention is directly linked to the kidneys' inability to effectively eliminate excess fluid from the body, a common phenomenon in patients suffering from chronic or acute renal failure.

In healthy kidneys, water and electrolytes are accurately filtered and reabsorbed, maintaining a stable water balance. However, when the kidneys fail to filter properly, excess water accumulates, leading to edema. These swellings are not only uncomfortable, they can also have serious consequences, such as difficulty in breathing (in the case of pulmonary edema), joint pain, or even aggravation of hypertension.

For a caregiver, it's crucial to regularly observe signs of edema, such as swollen legs or ankles, clothing or shoes that become too tight, or a rapid increase in body weight. Palpation can also reveal areas of skin that retain traces of prolonged pressure (bucket sign). Early detection of oedema enables care to be adapted rapidly, whether by adjusting the fluid balance, administering diuretics, or reinforcing clinical monitoring.

Hypotension: a drop in blood pressure

Hypotension, or low blood pressure, is a common phenomenon in dialysis patients, but can also occur in those with advanced renal dysfunction. During a hemodialysis session, excess fluid volume is removed from the bloodstream, which can sometimes lead to a too-rapid drop in blood pressure. This is often due to an excessive reduction in blood volume, rapid sodium loss, or maladaptation of the vascular system.

Symptoms of hypotension include dizziness, weakness, nausea, cold sweats and, in extreme cases, fainting. Hypotension is of particular concern because it can lead to inadequate perfusion of vital organs, especially the kidneys and brain, worsening the patient's condition.

For a caregiver, monitoring blood pressure before, during and after dialysis sessions is essential to prevent hypotension. If a drop in blood pressure is detected, it's crucial to react quickly, either by lying the patient down and raising the legs to improve venous return, or by slowing down the dialysis process or administering medically prescribed saline solutions to restore blood volume. The caregiver's vigilance is essential to prevent complications linked to hypotension, particularly in the most fragile patients.

Anuria: the absence of urine production

Anuria, or total absence of urine production, is an alarming sign of severe kidney failure. In a normal state, the kidneys continuously filter blood to produce urine, which eliminates waste products and excess fluids. However, in the case of anuria, the kidneys are no longer able to perform this function, leading to an accumulation of toxins and fluids in the body.

59

Anuria often occurs in the advanced stages of acute or chronic renal failure, or in cases of urinary tract obstruction. It can also be triggered by episodes of severe dehydration, hemodynamic shock, or conditions such as glomerulonephritis. The absence of urine production is a critical signal, as it indicates that the body is no longer eliminating its waste products and excess fluids, rapidly increasing the risk of water overload and metabolic intoxication.

In practice, caregivers need to keep a close eye on patients' diuresis and be able to recognize anuria. A patient who fails to produce urine for several hours or an entire day requires urgent medical assessment. In such situations, the use of replacement therapies, such as dialysis, becomes essential to replace failing renal function and avoid potentially fatal complications.

Hyperkalemia: excess potassium in the blood

Hyperkalemia, or elevated potassium levels in the blood, is one of the most dreaded complications of kidney failure. Potassium is an essential electrolyte for muscle and nervous system function, but excess can lead to serious disturbances, particularly in the heart. Normally, the kidneys eliminate excess potassium through urine, but when kidney function is impaired, potassium accumulates in the blood.

Hyperkalemia may be asymptomatic at first, but when it reaches dangerous levels, it manifests itself in clinical signs such as palpitations, muscle weakness, tingling, or heart rhythm disturbances, which can progress to severe arrhythmia and lead to cardiac arrest. This complication is particularly frequent in dialysis patients, or those whose diet is rich in potassium (such as fruit, green vegetables or legumes).

For a caregiver, vigilance against the risk of hyperkalemia is essential. He or she must ensure that patients comply with potassium dietary restrictions, monitor blood test results, and immediately report any suspicious signs, such as changes in heart rate or muscle cramps. When hyperkalemia is detected, prompt medical intervention is required, with treatments such as calcium to protect the heart, chelating resins to remove potassium, or emergency dialysis.

- **The importance of blood and urine tests**: Understanding common results (creatinine, urea, electrolytes).

Understanding common laboratory test results, such as creatinine, urea and electrolytes, is fundamental to monitoring patients with kidney disease. These biological parameters provide valuable information on renal function and the body's internal equilibrium. For a nephrology caregiver, knowing the significance of these results helps to better understand the patient's clinical condition, anticipate potential complications and collaborate effectively with the care team.

Creatinine: a key indicator of renal function

Creatinine is one of the most widely used markers of kidney function. It is a waste product of normal muscle metabolism, normally filtered and eliminated by the kidneys. The level of creatinine in the blood is directly related to the kidneys' ability to filter the blood: the more impaired the kidney function, the more creatinine accumulates in the blood.

In a healthy person, the kidneys efficiently filter creatinine, keeping blood levels low and constant. However, in patients with renal failure, creatinine levels rise progressively, reflecting a decrease in the kidneys' ability to eliminate this waste product. Elevated creatinine levels may therefore be a sign of acute or chronic renal deterioration.

Creatinine measurement is also used to calculate glomerular filtration rate (GFR), a key indicator of renal function. A low GFR indicates advanced renal failure, often requiring specific management, such as dialysis. For a caregiver, it's essential to understand that high creatinine values may require adaptations to care, such as closer monitoring or adjustments to medication regimens.

Urea: a reflection of nitrogen waste elimination

Urea is another important marker of renal function. It is produced in the liver during protein metabolism and then eliminated by the kidneys. Like creatinine, urea is a waste product that accumulates in the blood when the kidneys are not functioning properly. However, urea is a less specific indicator of kidney function, as its levels can also be influenced by other factors, such as diet (particularly a high-protein diet) or the patient's state of hydration.

In chronic kidney disease, an increase in urea in the blood, known as uraemia, is a sign that the kidneys are no longer able to eliminate nitrogen waste efficiently. This can lead to progressive intoxication of the body, with symptoms such as nausea, vomiting, itching and intense fatigue. In advanced cases, uraemia can lead to neurological or cardiovascular complications.

The caregiver should be aware that high urea levels may signal the need for urgent management, including dialysis to eliminate accumulated waste. It is also important to watch for clinical signs of uremia, such as digestive disturbances or lethargy, which should be reported to the medical team.

Electrolytes: maintaining water and electrolyte balance

Electrolytes, such as sodium, potassium and chloride, are essential for water balance, nerve transmission and muscle contraction. The kidneys play a key role in regulating these electrolytes, adjusting their concentration in the blood to the body's needs. When the kidneys fail, this balance is disturbed, with potentially serious consequences.

Sodium is the most abundant electrolyte in the blood and plays an essential role in regulating blood pressure and water balance. An abnormal concentration of sodium in the blood can be a sign of fluid imbalance. For example, hyponatremia (low sodium levels) may be linked to excessive water retention, often seen in patients with renal failure, while hypernatremia (high sodium levels) may indicate severe dehydration. These imbalances can lead to neurological symptoms such as headaches, confusion, or even convulsions in extreme cases.

Potassium is another essential electrolyte, mainly involved in muscle and heart function. In kidney failure, the kidneys are no longer able to excrete potassium properly, which can lead to hyperkalemia, an excess of potassium in the blood. Hyperkalemia is particularly dangerous, as it can lead to life-threatening cardiac arrhythmias. Patients with hyperkalemia may experience palpitations, muscle weakness or tingling. It's crucial for the caregiver to monitor these signs and ensure that patients respect their potassium dietary restrictions.

Chloride, another electrolyte regulated by the kidneys, helps maintain acid-base balance. Chloride imbalances may reflect disorders of overall electrolyte balance, or respiratory or metabolic problems. Hypochloremia (low chloride levels) may accompany sodium imbalances, while hyperchloremia (high chloride levels) is often associated with metabolic acidosis, an acid-base imbalance frequently seen in patients with renal failure.

Interpretation and clinical vigilance

Although these biological results are mainly analyzed by doctors and nurses, the caregiver must be able to understand their general significance and implications for the patient. For example, abnormal levels of creatinine, urea or electrolytes should prompt extra vigilance in monitoring clinical signs. A patient with hyperkalemia may rapidly develop cardiac complications, while elevated urea or creatinine may necessitate a change in care, such as adjustment of diuretic therapy or more frequent recourse to dialysis.

Careful monitoring of the clinical signs associated with these biological results is essential. Regular monitoring of blood pressure, weight and diuresis, **as** well as observation of symptoms such as edema, muscle cramps, nausea or mental confusion, can help detect imbalances early and avoid serious complications.

- **The caregiver's role in clinical observation**: noting subtle changes in the patient's condition.

Noting subtle changes in a patient's condition is a key skill for any healthcare professional, and it takes on particular importance in a nephrology department where patients are often faced with complex chronic pathologies. These small changes, which may seem insignificant at first glance, are often early warning signs of a deteriorating clinical condition or metabolic imbalance. As a caregiver, observing and reporting these subtle changes enables you to act quickly, prevent serious complications and ensure optimal care.

Daily vigilance in patient observation

Patients with kidney disease, whether on dialysis or being monitored for chronic renal failure, are likely to experience symptoms that evolve slowly and inconspicuously. Slightly increased fatigue, a change in appetite, or even a subtle variation in skin color may go unnoticed, but may reveal important underlying problems. As a caregiver, being alert to these slight changes is essential, as they are often the first signs that the patient's condition is changing.

Daily monitoring of the patient is based on continuous, in-depth observation of his or her physical appearance, behaviours and reactions. For example, a patient who suddenly becomes more listless or less interactive may indicate malaise, increased fatigue or a metabolic complication such as toxin accumulation. Slight swelling of the legs, hands or face may signal fluid retention, a sign of heart failure or fluid overload in dialysis patients. Similarly, discrete variations in skin color, such as paleness or slight yellowing, may indicate an imbalance in toxin elimination or anemia.

Physical signs to watch out for

One of the caregiver's first responsibilities is to note any physical changes in the patient's appearance. This includes changes in the skin, such as redness, signs of dehydration, or rashes. Skin texture may also change, becoming drier or scaly in patients suffering from electrolyte imbalances. These alterations may seem minor, but they should be reported promptly, as they may indicate a potential complication, particularly in relation to renal function.

Even slight swelling should also be carefully observed. If a patient has slight swelling in the ankles or feet, this may indicate fluid retention that was not present in previous days. These small changes are particularly important in dialysis patients, where fluid management is crucial to avoid cardiovascular and pulmonary complications. A subtle increase in weight between two dialysis sessions can also reveal fluid overload, necessitating adjustment of treatment.

Behavioral and emotional signs

In addition to physical changes, behavioral or emotional changes can be key indicators of a patient's state of health. A normally alert and communicative patient who becomes more tired, irritable or confused may be suffering from an accumulation of toxins in the blood, a common phenomenon in advanced renal failure. Symptoms such as lethargy or episodes of mental confusion may indicate uraemia (urea accumulation) or uraemic encephalopathy, which require prompt management.

Another example is decreased appetite, which is often an early sign of metabolic imbalances. If a patient starts eating less or complaining of nausea, this may indicate a retention of toxic waste in the blood. By noting this subtle change, the caregiver can alert nurses or doctors to the problem, who can then check whether biological parameters, such as urea or creatinine, are rising dangerously high.

Monitoring vital signs

In addition to physical and behavioral observations, vital signs provide a valuable indicator of subtle changes in the patient's condition. A slight increase in blood pressure may indicate fluid retention or electrolyte imbalance, while sudden hypotension may signal dehydration or a complication during a dialysis session.

Temperature readings should also be carefully monitored. A slight fever may go unnoticed, but it can be an early sign of infection, particularly in patients with catheters or fistulas. Caregivers must therefore be vigilant and record every temperature fluctuation, however slight, as an untreated infection can quickly become complicated in a patient already weakened by renal failure.

The importance of communication with the care team

Caregivers' observations, though seemingly straightforward, play a central role in patient care. Indeed, caregivers often spend the most time with patients, and are in the front line of observing subtle changes. Regular and effective communication with nurses and doctors is therefore essential if this information is to be taken into account in clinical decisions.

For example, if a caregiver notices that the patient is becoming increasingly fatigued, has mild edema or decreased diuresis, these observations may lead to a reassessment of fluid management or adjustments to diuretic therapy. Similarly, careful observation of eating habits or changes in pain management can help identify complications more quickly, enabling early intervention.

Chapter 5

Supporting dialysis patients

- **Understanding dialysis: hemodialysis and peritoneal dialysis**: principle, operation and differences.

Principle, function and differences are fundamental aspects to understand when comparing different methods or technologies, particularly in nephrology where these concepts apply to treatments such as hemodialysis and peritoneal dialysis. Understanding these notions not only enables you to grasp the basics of medical procedures, but also to identify why some treatments are better suited to certain patients than others.

Principle: the theoretical basis that guides a method

The principle of a treatment or technology refers to the concept or theory on which it is based. In nephrology, the principle of dialysis, for example, is simple: to replace failing kidney function by removing waste products and excess fluid from the blood when the kidneys can no longer do so. It's a method of kidney replacement that artificially reproduces one of the kidneys' main functions: blood filtration.

In hemodialysis, the principle is based on the use of a machine that filters blood through a semi-permeable membrane to eliminate toxins, excess salts and water. For peritoneal dialysis, the principle is similar, but instead of using an external machine, the peritoneum, a natural membrane located in the abdomen, acts as a filter. Both methods share the same fundamental objective: to purify the blood and maintain electrolyte balance, but they differ in the way they achieve this goal.

Operation: the concrete process that implements the principle

How a treatment works explains how this principle is applied in practice. In hemodialysis, the patient's blood is removed from the body through a vascular access device, such as an arteriovenous fistula, and passed into a dialyzer, or "artificial kidney". This dialyzer contains a semi-permeable membrane that allows small molecules (such as urea, potassium and excess fluid) to pass from the blood into a dialysis fluid on the other side of the membrane. After filtration, the purified blood is returned to the body. This process generally takes place over a period of 4 to 5 hours, three times a week, in a dialysis center or at home, depending on the patient's capabilities and medical protocols.

Peritoneal dialysis works in a slightly different way. Here, a catheter is surgically implanted in the patient's abdominal cavity. A sterile liquid, called dialysate, is introduced into the abdomen through this catheter. The dialysate comes into contact with the peritoneum, which acts as a natural membrane for filtering waste and excess fluids from the blood. After a few hours, this toxin-containing fluid is drained from the abdomen and replaced by a new dialysis solution. This process is less time-consuming and can be carried out at home, either manually several times a day (ambulatory peritoneal dialysis), or automatically during the night (automated peritoneal dialysis).

Differences: variations between methods and their impact on the patient

The differences between hemodialysis and peritoneal dialysis mainly concern the method used, the setting in which it is performed, the patient's needs and the associated risks. These differences are important in choosing the treatment best suited to each patient's lifestyle, state of health and personal preferences.

Hemodialysis is a more invasive method, requiring the creation of a vascular access and the use of an external machine to filter the blood. It is generally carried out in a dialysis center, under the supervision of healthcare professionals, although some patients may undergo it at home. It requires regular attendance at the center, often three times a week, which can be restrictive for patients in terms of mobility and lifestyle flexibility. Hemodialysis is also associated with abrupt variations in fluid and electrolyte balance, which can lead to side effects such as cramps, hypotension or headaches.

Peritoneal dialysis, on the other hand, is generally gentler and can be performed at home, offering greater freedom and flexibility to the patient. Peritoneal dialysis is continuous, allowing more stable fluid and toxin management, without the abrupt fluctuations sometimes seen with hemodialysis. However, peritoneal dialysis carries specific risks, notably catheter or peritoneal cavity infections (peritonitis), which can be serious. This method is also less suitable for patients who have already undergone several abdominal operations, or whose peritoneum is not functioning properly.

Another notable difference lies in time management and autonomy. Hemodialysis, though effective, imposes a rigid rhythm and requires a specific infrastructure. Peritoneal dialysis, on the other hand, enables patients to be more autonomous, carrying out their treatments at home, with the possibility of adapting their schedule to suit their needs.

- **Prepare a patient for a dialysis session**: reassure, check fistula status, manage equipment.

As part of the management of hemodialysis patients, reassuring the patient, checking the condition of the arteriovenous fistula, and managing the equipment are essential steps in ensuring the safety and efficacy of the treatment, and the well-being of the patient. Hemodialysis is a regular treatment, often perceived as stressful by patients due to its invasive nature and the dependency it engenders. The role of the caregiver is therefore vital in creating a serene environment, ensuring that the patient and equipment are properly prepared, and preventing complications.

Reassuring the patient: creating a climate of trust and serenity

For many patients, each hemodialysis session can be a source of anxiety, especially as it involves the use of a vascular access that can seem impressive and potentially painful. Reassuring the patient is therefore a fundamental step, both emotionally and physically. It is essential to adopt an empathetic approach, to take the time to listen to the patient's concerns, and to answer his or her questions clearly and sympathetically. A reassured patient will be more relaxed, making treatment easier and more comfortable during the session.

Fear of pain or fistula-related complications is an aspect often raised by patients. The caregiver can explain, step by step, how the procedure will be carried out, emphasizing the measures taken to minimize discomfort and avoid risks. This moment of dialogue helps to build confidence and alleviate patient anxiety, which is particularly important for people who experience these sessions repeatedly and often tiringly.

Checking the condition of the arteriovenous fistula: a crucial safety step

The arteriovenous fistula, which connects an artery to a vein, is the preferred vascular access for hemodialysis, due to its reliability and longevity. However, this access requires constant vigilance, as complications such as infection, thrombosis or stenosis (narrowing of the vessels) can occur. Before each dialysis session, the dialysis assistant must carry out a thorough check of the fistula to ensure that it is in good working order.

Checking the condition of the fistula begins with visual observation: this involves checking for signs of infection, such as redness, swelling or unusual discharge around the access area. Next, the caregiver must gently palpate the fistula to ensure that there is a vibration, called a "thrill", which is a sign that blood flow is correct. If this vibration is absent or abnormal, it may indicate a blood circulation problem, and medical intervention should be considered. Auscultation with a stethoscope can also confirm the presence of a "noise" (murmur), an audible sign of normal blood flow through the fistula.

Proper monitoring of the fistula is essential to prevent serious complications such as thrombosis, which can compromise vascular access and require emergency surgery. What's more, a fistula in poor condition can render the dialysis session ineffective, with a direct impact on the patient's health.

Material management: ensuring rigorous preparation

Material management is another crucial responsibility for the caregiver when preparing a hemodialysis session. The smooth running of dialysis depends on meticulous organization and rigorous hygiene, as the risk of infection is always present due to the invasive nature of the treatment.

Equipment preparation begins with a check of the dialysis machine, which must be precisely set according to patient-specific parameters (such as session duration, volume of fluid to be removed, and filtration rates). The caregiver must ensure that all necessary equipment is sterile, especially the needles used to insert the fistula. Adherence to disinfection protocols is essential to avoid infection, notably by carefully cleaning the access area before placing the needles.

Needle management for fistula puncture is a delicate task, as improper handling can cause pain, bleeding or damage to the vascular access. Needles must be precisely placed to allow good blood flow to the machine, without traumatizing the blood vessels. The caregiver must also be attentive to patient monitoring during the dialysis session: in the event of blood leakage or discomfort, rapid intervention is required to adjust the equipment or reposition the needles.

After the session, equipment management doesn't stop. The caregiver must ensure that everything is properly disinfected, that used needles are disposed of according to safety protocols, and that the machine is cleaned and ready for the next use. Good equipment management is not only a question of safety, but also of efficiency, since an error or defect in the equipment can compromise the patient's treatment.

- **Assist during the session**: monitor vital parameters, prevent complications (hypotension, cramps).

Monitoring vital parameters and preventing complications such as hypotension and cramps are essential aspects of hemodialysis patient management. Dialysis, because of its invasive nature and direct impact on the body's water and electrolyte balance, requires continuous attention to ensure the patient's safety and well-being. The caregiver plays a crucial role in this monitoring, observing the patient's clinical signs throughout the session and acting quickly to prevent or manage complications.

Monitoring vital parameters: regular follow-up to anticipate risks

Monitoring vital parameters such as blood pressure, heart rate and temperature is essential to assess the patient's condition during a hemodialysis session. Each patient reacts differently to dialysis, depending on his or her state of health, fluid balance and cardiac condition. It is therefore essential to monitor these indicators throughout the session to detect any subtle changes that could signal an imbalance or complication.

Blood pressure is probably the most important parameter to monitor during dialysis. Indeed, the rapid reduction in blood volume due to fluid elimination can lead to a drop in blood pressure (hypotension). Before the session, a blood pressure reading is taken to assess the patient's initial condition and determine whether he or she is ready to start dialysis. During the session, regular blood pressure readings, often every 15 to 30 minutes, are taken to check that the body is tolerating the

75

elimination of fluids. If the pressure drops abruptly, signs such as dizziness, nausea or cold sweats may appear. The caregiver must then intervene quickly to adjust the patient's position (by lying down with legs elevated) or alert the medical team to reduce the filtration rate or administer saline solutions.

Heart rate is also monitored for signs of cardiac overexertion, particularly in patients with a previous history of heart disease. Tachycardia (rapid increase in heart rate) may indicate overexertion of the heart to compensate for hypotension or fluid overload, while bradycardia (slowing of the heart) could signal vasovagal malaise or another complication associated with hemodialysis.

Temperature is another parameter to monitor, although it is less directly related to dialysis itself. However, a slight rise in temperature can be an early sign of infection, particularly if the patient uses a catheter for dialysis, or if bacteria have penetrated through the vascular access. Regular temperature monitoring, especially after the session, can detect these signs and act quickly to prevent possible sepsis.

Preventing hypotension: anticipate and react quickly

Hypotension is one of the most frequent complications of hemodialysis. It occurs when the body fails to adapt to the rapid loss of fluid during the session. This drop in blood pressure can lead to uncomfortable and sometimes dangerous symptoms, such as dizziness, nausea, paleness, or loss of consciousness in the most serious cases.

To prevent this complication, the caregiver must not only monitor vital parameters, but also be alert to the warning signs of hypotension. The **patient's weight** before the session is a key indicator: excessive weight gain between two dialysis sessions suggests an excessive accumulation of fluids, thus increasing the risk of hypotension when these fluids are rapidly eliminated. Monitoring weight therefore helps determine the amount of fluid to be removed during the session, a crucial parameter in avoiding excessive dehydration.

The caregiver's role is also to ensure that the patient is properly hydrated before dialysis, without exceeding set limits. Advice on managing fluid intake between sessions can also be given to help prevent excessive fluid overload, often responsible for hypotension.

In the event of a drop in blood pressure during dialysis, the first intervention is usually to **modify the patient's position**, by placing him or her in dorsal decubitus (lying on his or her back) with legs elevated. This promotes venous return and can help stabilize blood pressure. If hypotension persists, a saline solution can be administered to restore blood volume.

Preventing cramps: managing fluid and electrolyte balance

Muscle cramps, particularly in the legs, are another common complication of hemodialysis. They often occur as a result of **rapid fluid loss** or electrolyte imbalance during blood filtration. When muscles lack fluid or certain electrolytes, such as sodium or potassium, they can contract involuntarily, causing intense pain and discomfort for the patient.

To prevent cramps, careful monitoring of **fluid balance** is essential. If too much fluid is withdrawn too quickly, muscles can become dehydrated, increasing the risk of cramps. By adjusting the filtration rate and ensuring that the volume of fluid withdrawn is not exceeded, the caregiver and medical team can limit this risk. **Monitoring electrolytes** in the blood before the session is also crucial to anticipate imbalances and adapt treatments if necessary.

If a patient experiences cramping during the session, a first intervention is to adjust the dialysis speed to reduce the rate of fluid withdrawal. Gentle stretching exercises can also be suggested to relieve the affected muscles. Sometimes, specific dietary supplements or dietary adjustments may be recommended to help maintain a better electrolyte balance.

Chapter 6

Nutrition and hydration in nephrology patients

- **The importance of diet in renal failure**: a diet low in sodium, potassium and phosphorus.

A diet low in sodium, potassium and phosphorus is an essential component in the management of patients with kidney disease. When the kidneys no longer function properly, they can no longer effectively eliminate excesses of these minerals, which can lead to serious imbalances in the body, affecting the heart, bones and other vital systems. Adopting such a diet can limit these imbalances, reduce the progression of kidney disease, and improve patients' quality of life. However, this type of diet requires particular vigilance, both in terms of food choices and the quantity of food consumed, as these minerals are found in many everyday products.

Sodium: limiting water retention and hypertension

Sodium, found mainly in table salt, plays a key role in regulating water balance and blood pressure. When the kidneys fail, their ability to eliminate sodium is impaired, leading to an accumulation of sodium in the body. This accumulation causes water retention, aggravating hypertension and edema (swelling), and increasing the risk of cardiac overload. A low-sodium diet therefore aims to reduce salt consumption to prevent these complications.

Patients with kidney disease need to pay particular attention to **hidden sources of sodium** in processed foods, such as ready-made meals, deli meats, industrial sauces and salty snacks. Even foods that don't seem salty can contain significant amounts of sodium, such as industrial breads and cereals. It is often advisable to cook without adding salt, and to replace salty condiments with spices, fresh herbs or lemon juice to add flavour without increasing sodium intake.

Compliance with this restriction is crucial, as high sodium intake can rapidly worsen a kidney patient's condition, especially if he or she is on dialysis or suffering from heart failure. Specific dietary advice is often provided by a dietician to help the patient identify sodium-rich foods and make the best food choices.

Potassium: preventing heart complications

Potassium is an essential mineral for muscle and nerve function, and in particular for regulating the heartbeat. However, in patients with kidney disease, the inability of the kidneys to remove excess potassium from the blood can lead to hyperkalemia (high potassium levels), which is dangerous because it can cause heart rhythm disturbances and even cardiac arrest.

To prevent these complications, patients should follow a -low potassium **diet**, limiting consumption of foods naturally rich in this mineral. These foods include many fruits and vegetables, such as bananas, oranges, potatoes, tomatoes and spinach. This can make the application of this diet particularly restrictive, as these foods are often considered healthy, but become harmful to kidney patients when consumed in excess.

However, food preparation methods can help reduce potassium levels. For example, we recommend **boiling vegetables** (such as potatoes or carrots) and discarding the cooking water, as some of the potassium is eliminated in the water. Some fruits can be replaced by low-potassium options, such as apples, berries or pears. The support of a dietician is essential to ensure adequate nutritional intake while avoiding the risk of hyperkalemia.

Phosphorus: maintaining healthy bones and vessels

Phosphorus is a mineral necessary for healthy bones and teeth, but when the kidneys can no longer eliminate it properly, it accumulates in the blood, leading to abnormal calcium and phosphorus levels. This imbalance can lead to calcium deposits in blood vessels, joints and organs, increasing the risk of cardiovascular disease, joint pain and renal osteodystrophy (brittle bones).

To avoid these complications, a **low-phosphorus diet** is recommended, which involves reducing consumption of certain phosphorus-rich foods, such as dairy products (milk, cheeses), processed meats, fatty fish, nuts, legumes and cola-based drinks. These foods are often high in protein, which can make it difficult to balance the patient's nutritional needs with the need to limit phosphorus.

Patients should also be aware of phosphorus-rich **food additives**, often found in processed foods and soft drinks. These additives are generally used as preservatives or to improve the texture of products, but they can considerably increase phosphorus intake without this being immediately visible on labels.

In addition to a low-phosphorus diet, patients may be prescribed **phosphorus binders**, drugs that bind to phosphorus in the intestines and prevent it from being absorbed into the bloodstream. To be effective, these drugs must be taken with meals. Phosphorus management is particularly important for preserving long-term bone health and preventing vascular calcification.

- **The caregiver's involvement in food monitoring**: adapting meal trays, monitoring water intake.

Adapting meal plans and monitoring fluid intake are two crucial elements in the management of patients suffering from kidney disease. These dietary adjustments aim to prevent complications linked to mineral and fluid imbalances, while taking into account the specific restrictions of each patient. For a caregiver, it is essential to understand the principles guiding these adaptations and to rigorously monitor the patient's diet and water consumption, in collaboration with the medical team and dieticians.

Adapting meal trays: meeting nutritional needs while respecting restrictions

Adapting meal trays for patients with kidney disease is essential to ensure a balanced diet, while respecting the many dietary restrictions that accompany this type of pathology. Renal failure patients often have to follow specific diets, low in sodium, potassium, phosphorus, and sometimes protein, depending on the progression of their disease. Adapting meals not only means reducing or eliminating certain foods, but also ensuring that meals are appetizing and varied, to encourage patients to eat enough despite the restrictions.

In a **low-sodium** diet, for example, it's crucial to avoid salt-rich foods such as deli meats, ready-made meals, canned goods and industrial condiments. Instead, meals should be prepared from fresh ingredients, using herbs, mild spices and salt-free alternatives to enhance flavors. Foods high in **potassium**, such as bananas, potatoes or tomatoes, should also be limited, and it is sometimes necessary to favor specific cooking techniques, such as boiling vegetables and discarding the cooking water to reduce their potassium content.

In addition, the adaptation of meal trays must take into account **phosphorus** limitation, a mineral found in dairy products, processed meats, fatty fish and many processed foods. Replacing these products with low-phosphorus foods, such as certain types of fruit and vegetables, and adding high-quality proteins in controlled quantities (such as egg whites or lean meats), enables nutritional requirements to be met without overloading the kidneys.

Finally, the psychological aspect must not be overlooked. It's important to keep meals attractive and varied, despite restrictions, to encourage patients to eat well. Monotonous or insipid meals can discourage patients, and lead to malnutrition, a frequent problem among people with chronic illnesses. Assistance from a dietician is often essential to design meals that combine pleasure and health, while respecting the limits imposed by the pathology.

Monitoring water intake: a delicate balance to avoid overload or dehydration

Managing fluid intake in patients with kidney disease is an ongoing challenge, particularly in those with advanced renal failure or on dialysis. The kidneys can no longer effectively eliminate excess fluid, which can lead to a build-up of water in the body, causing edema, hypertension and heart or lung complications. To avoid these complications, it is essential to limit water intake, while ensuring that patients do not suffer from dehydration.

The **amount of fluid** allowed per day depends on the patient's condition and the amount of urine he or she produces. For some patients on dialysis, intake may be limited to around 500 to 1000 millilitres a day, depending on the amount of residual fluid their kidneys can eliminate. This includes not only water and beverages, but also liquids contained in foods such as soups, juicy fruits (like melons or oranges), and ice creams. Strict monitoring of these intakes is necessary to avoid fluid overload, which can lead to serious complications such as pulmonary edema or heart failure.

The caregiver must therefore ensure that the amount of fluids consumed is strictly controlled. This includes ensuring that the patient complies with the daily drinking recommendations, by providing small amounts of water regularly rather than large quantities at a time, to better distribute water intake over the day. Tips such as using small cups or tumblers can also help avoid excessive consumption. In addition, it's essential to explain the reasons for these restrictions to the patient, in order to gain his or her support and prevent thirst-related frustrations, which can be intense.

In some cases, **managing thirst** can be a real challenge, especially for patients who experience excessive thirst as a result of their diet or medication. To help control this sensation, alternatives such as chewing on ice cubes, rinsing the mouth with cool water without swallowing, or eating fruits rich in water but low in potassium, such as apples or pears in small quantities, can be suggested.

Weight monitoring is another key method of monitoring a patient's fluid balance. Rapid weight gain between dialysis sessions is often a sign of fluid retention. Every day, the patient's weight should be measured, ideally at the same time of day, to check that he or she is not gaining excessive weight due to water overload. A sudden increase in weight should be reported to the medical team, as it may indicate that water intake is too high, or that dialysis is not sufficiently effective.

- **Support for controlled hydration**: Calculation and monitoring of water balance as prescribed.

Calculating and monitoring fluid balance as prescribed are essential steps in the management of patients with kidney disease, particularly those with acute or advanced chronic renal failure. These patients have a reduced capacity to eliminate fluids, which can lead to an accumulation of water in the body, causing edema, hypertension and other serious complications such as pulmonary edema or heart failure. Water balance monitoring consists of comparing fluid intake and losses (particularly diuresis) to maintain an optimal balance, and thus avoid water overload or dehydration. Compliance with medical prescriptions is crucial to ensure effective fluid management.

Calculating the water balance: understanding the concept and its importance

Fluid balance is the difference between fluid intake and fluid loss. It is used to assess whether the patient is eliminating sufficient fluids to compensate for those consumed. In patients with renal failure, the kidneys are no longer able to eliminate excess fluid efficiently, which can lead to water retention. Conversely, excessive elimination without sufficient intake can lead to dehydration. Monitoring this balance is therefore essential to adjust care and avoid dangerous imbalances.

To calculate the fluid balance, you first need to account for **fluid intake**, which includes not only water and beverages consumed, but also fluids present in foods (such as soups and water-rich fruits) and those administered intravenously (infusions). Next, it is necessary to measure **fluid losses**, mainly diuresis (the amount of urine produced), but also other less visible losses, such as vomiting, diarrhea, or insensible losses linked to sweating and breathing.

Calculating the water balance is very simple: the body's losses are subtracted from its water intake. A **positive fluid balance** means that the patient is accumulating more fluid than he or she is eliminating, which can lead to fluid overload. Conversely, a **negative water balance** indicates that losses are greater than intakes, which can lead to dehydration.

Monitoring fluid intake: comply with medical prescriptions

In renal patients, water intake is often strictly limited according to the residual capacity of the kidneys to eliminate water. Medical prescriptions vary according to the volume of urine produced (if any), the patient's general condition and activity level. For example, a dialysis patient may be limited to a water intake of 500 to 1000 millilitres per day, including water, beverages and liquid foods.

The nursing auxiliary plays an essential role in **rigorously monitoring fluid intake**. He or she must ensure that the patient does not exceed the prescribed amount of fluid, even if the sensation of thirst is intense, which can be difficult for patients to manage. This involves meticulously counting every glass of water, every cup of coffee, or every serving of soup, and recording them so as not to exceed the set limit. Little tricks, such as offering to chew ice cubes or using small cups to divide up the intake, can help to keep to these restrictions without causing too much frustration for the patient.

Monitoring water loss: measure and record diuresis

Measuring **diuresis** (urine production) is the main method of monitoring water loss. In renal patients, the amount of urine produced may be very low (oliguria) or even non-existent (anuria), reflecting the severity of renal failure. Diuresis is measured over a 24-hour period for accurate assessment. Each micturition is collected and accurately measured to calculate the total amount of urine produced during the day.

When the patient is on dialysis, it is also important to measure the amount of fluid removed by the machine during the session. This is part of **fluid loss**, and is crucial for adjusting intake between sessions. If dialysis has removed a large amount of fluid, fluid intake can sometimes be increased slightly under medical supervision, but any imbalance must be avoided.

Other losses, such as vomiting or diarrhea, must also be accounted for, as they can lead to significant losses of water and electrolytes. The caregiver should monitor any episodes of vomiting or diarrhoea and record the approximate amount of fluid lost.

Adapt care to water balance

Once the water balance has been calculated, it is important to analyze it in relation to the patient's condition and therapeutic objectives. A **positive fluid balance** may indicate fluid overload, signaled by symptoms such as edema (swelling), shortness of breath, or rapid weight gain. In such cases, corrective measures are often required, such as reducing fluid intake, adjusting diuretic therapy, or performing dialysis to eliminate excess fluid.

Conversely, a **negative water balance** can be a sign of dehydration. Symptoms include dry mouth, low blood pressure, increased fatigue, and sometimes dizziness. In such cases, a reassessment of fluid intake is necessary to rehydrate the patient in a controlled manner.

By accurately recording intake and output, and reporting any abnormalities to the medical team, the caregiver plays a key role in adapting care. Careful monitoring enables rapid reaction to the first signs of overload or dehydration, thus avoiding serious complications such as pulmonary edema or heart failure, which are major risks for renal patients.

Chapter 7

Psychological support for nephrology patients

- **The psychological impact of kidney disease**: stress, anxiety, depression.

Stress, anxiety and depression are common psychological reactions in patients with chronic illnesses such as kidney failure. These emotions stem from uncertainty, the constraints of treatment, and radical changes in lifestyle. These patients' daily lives are often punctuated by dialysis sessions, restrictive diets, and constant worry about the progression of their disease. Understanding and managing these psychological aspects is essential, as mental well-being directly influences disease management and quality of life.

Stress: the daily pressure of treatment and uncertainty

Stress is often linked to managing the physical and emotional constraints imposed by kidney disease. Treatment, particularly dialysis, requires strict discipline, regular hospital visits, and strict adherence to dietary and water restrictions. This creates constant pressure on the patient, who must not only adapt to these demands but also cope with the potential side effects of treatment, such as fatigue, cramps or low blood pressure.

Stress can also stem from uncertainty about the evolution of the disease. Patients are often faced with the anguish of not knowing whether their condition will stabilize, worsen, or whether they will ever need to consider a transplant. This feeling of unpredictability creates a permanent tension, where each new analysis or consultation becomes a source of stress. Some patients also feel social pressure, as they have to adjust their daily, professional or family activities to the demands of their treatment.

Stress management is therefore crucial to maintaining emotional balance. It is important for caregivers to recognize signs of stress, such as excessive fatigue, irritability or sleep disturbances, and to offer support, whether through reassuring discussions, the use of relaxation techniques, or referral to a psychologist.

Anxiety: the constant fear of deteriorating health

Anxiety, on the other hand, goes beyond everyday stress. It's a deeper, more persistent form of worry, often associated with irrational or exaggerated fears. In kidney patients, this anxiety can manifest itself as a constant fear of deteriorating health, the possibility of a sudden complication, or the possibility of not being eligible for a transplant. This fear is fuelled by the chronic, incurable nature of kidney failure, which places patients in a state of constant vigilance, always fearing the worst.

Dialysis sessions themselves can be a source of anxiety. For some patients, the idea of being dependent on a machine for survival is deeply distressing. Others dread possible complications during dialysis, such as hypotension or cramps, or possible infections linked to vascular access. Added to this is the fear of losing more autonomy, of having to limit their activities or social interactions even further.

Anxiety manifests itself through physical symptoms such as palpitations, tremors, excessive sweating, and sometimes panic attacks. Psychologically, patients may feel nervous, tense or unable to relax. Emotional support is essential to alleviate these anxieties. Caregivers, especially orderlies who are in direct and regular contact with patients, play a fundamental role in creating a climate of trust and responding empathetically to questions and concerns. Sometimes, psychological or psychiatric follow-up may be necessary, the with help of a professional specialized in anxiety management.

Depression: loss of meaning and feelings of powerlessness

Depression is often the result of accumulated mental fatigue in the face of chronic illness. In kidney patients, depression often arises when the disease is experienced as an insurmountable burden. The idea of living with a heavy pathology, requiring lifelong treatment, can engender a profound sense of despair and discouragement. Patients may feel that they no longer have any control over their lives, that they are caught up in a spiral of care and constraints.

This feeling of helplessness is exacerbated by dependence on dialysis or constant medical care. Some patients become depressed at the thought that they will never be able to regain their autonomy or lead the life they had before the disease. Depression in these patients can manifest itself as withdrawal, loss of interest in activities previously enjoyed, lack of appetite, sleep disturbances, even suicidal thoughts.

Depression, if left untreated, can have a direct impact on adherence to treatment. A depressed patient may neglect their care, stop following their diet, or miss dialysis sessions, all of which can worsen their condition. It is therefore vital that caregivers are alert to signs of depression, such as apathy, permanent sadness, or disinterest in social interaction. Depression often requires a multidisciplinary approach, combining psychological support, possibly medication, and regular monitoring by healthcare professionals.

- **Supporting patients with chronic fatigue**: Listening and support techniques.

Listening and accompaniment techniques are essential to providing effective, caring support to patients, particularly in the nephrology setting, where care often goes beyond the medical aspect to encompass emotional support. Patients with chronic kidney disease face heavy treatments, such as dialysis, as well as major lifestyle changes. They may experience anxiety, stress, and feelings of uncertainty or loneliness. For these reasons, knowing how to listen actively and accompany patients with empathy and respect is crucial to promoting their psychological well-being, while facilitating their adherence to treatment.

Active listening: being fully present for the patient

Active listening is a fundamental technique in patient care. It involves paying attention to what the patient is expressing, not only in words, but also through behavior, tone of voice and emotions. Active listening goes beyond passive hearing; it involves an attentive attitude, an open posture, and responses that show the patient that he or she is heard and understood.

Being **fully present** for the patient is the first step towards active listening. This means avoiding distractions, such as consulting documents or interrupting the conversation. It's important to maintain friendly eye contact and adopt a non-judgmental posture that invites confidence. This approach creates a climate of trust, where patients feel safe to express their concerns, fears or doubts without fear of being misunderstood or ignored.

Specific active listening techniques include simple but powerful gestures, such as **nodding to** show that you're following what the patient is saying, or **short verbal responses** like "I see", "I understand", which confirm that the caregiver is paying attention. Asking **open-ended questions** encourages the patient to express himself or herself more fully, and gives a better idea of how he or she really feels. For example, instead of asking a closed question like "How are you?", it's more effective to ask: "How are you feeling today with your treatment?" This invites the patient to reflect and share deeper feelings.

Empathy: understanding the patient's emotions

Empathy is at the heart of successful support. It's the ability to put yourself in the patient's shoes, to understand their emotions and suffering, without being overwhelmed by them. In nephrology, patients are confronted with exhausting treatments and uncertainties about their future, which can generate anxiety, stress and even anger. Showing empathy helps to lighten this emotional load by acknowledging and validating the patient's feelings.

An empathetic response is not simply to say "I understand", but to rephrase what the patient is expressing to show them that their emotions are legitimate. For example, if a patient confides that he or she feels exhausted and discouraged by dialysis, an empathetic response might be, "I can see that dialysis sessions are very trying for you, it must be difficult to manage every week." This reformulation not only shows the patient that their emotions are being heard, but also encourages them to continue expressing how they feel, reinforcing the bond of trust.

Empathy also manifests itself in simple but meaningful **physical gestures**, such as a hand gently placed on the patient's shoulder or a kind smile, which bring comfort without the need for words. These small gestures humanize the caregiver-patient relationship and show that the professional is there not only to treat the illness, but also to support the whole person.

Validating emotions: recognizing without judging

One of the key techniques in support is **emotional validation**. This involves acknowledging the patient's feelings without minimizing or judging them. All too often, in the face of patient distress or frustration, caregivers may be tempted to reassure too quickly or rationalize emotions ("Don't worry, everything will be fine"). However, this can leave patients with the impression that their feelings are not being taken seriously.

Instead, validating the patient's emotions means welcoming them **without judgment**, whether they be sadness, anger or worry. For example, if a patient expresses frustration because they feel dependent on dialysis, instead of immediately responding with advice or solutions, it's important to acknowledge this feeling first: "I understand that this dependence on dialysis can be frustrating, it's a big adjustment to go through on a daily basis." This shows the patient that their feelings are normal and that their emotions are legitimate.

Emotional validation doesn't solve the problem, but it often calms the patient's mind by making them feel understood and supported, which may be enough to reduce some of their anxiety.

Supporting without directing: encouraging autonomy

Support does not always mean providing solutions or answers. It often means **guiding without directing**, i.e. encouraging patients to find their own solutions and make decisions about their health. This is particularly important in the case of chronic diseases such as kidney failure, where patients must learn to manage their treatment over the long term and adapt to new constraints.

Encouraging autonomy means asking open-ended questions that prompt patients to think about their own resources and choices. For example, instead of telling a patient what to do when faced with a difficulty, we can ask: "What solutions could help you better manage your fatigue after dialysis sessions?" This allows the patient to become actively involved in his or her own care, and reinforces his or her sense of control over the disease.

It's also important to help patients make decisions without overwhelming them with technical information or complex choices. The caregiver can, for example, propose simple, well-explained options, guiding the patient towards solutions while respecting his or her preferences and abilities.

Emotional support: being there for the long haul

Finally, support is not limited to a specific moment in time, but is a long-term process. Patients with chronic illnesses experience **emotional ups and downs**, and it's important for the caregiver to be available not only at times of crisis, but also on a daily basis. This means **regularly monitoring** the patient's emotional progress, checking on how they are feeling, and making sure they don't feel isolated or abandoned.

Emotional monitoring allows us to spot early signs of depression or heightened anxiety, and intervene before these problems become too much to handle. A simple "How are you feeling today?" or "Is there anything worrying you at the moment?" can open the door to important discussions, and offer the patient a space to express his or her concerns.

- **The helping relationship at the end of life or while waiting for a transplant**: Ethical and emotional support.

Ethical and emotional support is an essential component of nephrology care, where the human dimension is as important as medical care. Patients with chronic or end-stage kidney disease face considerable challenges, both physical and emotional. The suffering associated with progressive loss of autonomy, dependence on treatments such as dialysis, and uncertainties about the future often generate profound anxiety. In this context, support is not limited to simply managing medical symptoms, but also involves emotional support and consideration of ethical values that respect the patient's dignity and choices.

Ethical support: respecting patients' dignity and choices

Ethical support is based on fundamental principles that aim to respect patients' dignity, autonomy and rights. In nephrology care, these principles are essential, as patients are often faced with difficult decisions concerning their treatment, particularly with regard to hemodialysis, peritoneal dialysis or, in some cases, discontinuation of care. As a caregiver, it's crucial to ensure that every patient is treated with respect, and that their decisions are taken into account, even when they may seem contrary to medical expectations.

Patient autonomy is at the heart of ethical care. This means that every individual has the right to actively participate in decisions concerning his or her treatment and health. In situations where the patient has to choose between different therapeutic options, such as continuing dialysis or opting for palliative care, the role of the caregiver is to provide clear, objective information while respecting the patient's personal choices. It is essential to avoid any form of pressure or judgment, and to enable the patient to make informed decisions, in line with his or her values and conception of quality of life.

Another aspect of ethical care is confidentiality and respect for privacy. In a department as personal as nephrology, where patients often share intimate information about their health, it is essential that caregivers take care to protect this information and maintain a relationship of trust. Every exchange must be conducted with the utmost confidentiality, guaranteeing patients that their medical information is treated with the utmost care and shared only with those directly involved in their care.

Finally, ethical support also means taking into account the **limits of medical intervention**. Some patients, particularly those at the end of life or suffering from end-stage renal failure, may refuse treatments they consider too restrictive or of little benefit to them. Respecting this decision, even if it runs counter to therapeutic objectives, is an act of ethical support. It means accepting that, sometimes, comfort, quality of life and personal wishes take precedence over prolonging life at all costs. In this context, caregivers must ensure that care remains patient-centred, by listening to the patient's needs and encouraging open discussion of his or her expectations and wishes for the future.

Emotional support: providing empathetic, personalized support

Emotional support is just as important as the ethical aspect, providing patients with human and empathetic support in the face of the trials they are going through. Chronic kidney disease is often experienced as a progressive loss of control over one's body and life, generating feelings of frustration, anxiety and sometimes depression. Caregivers need to be able to recognize and manage these emotions, in order to improve the patient's psychological well-being.

The first step in emotional support is to **actively listen to** the patient. As mentioned above, active listening is a technique that involves being fully present for the patient, listening without judging, and allowing them to freely express their fears, doubts and suffering. Many patients, especially those facing invasive treatments such as dialysis, feel a profound sense of isolation and powerlessness. It is therefore essential to offer them a safe space where they can confide and share their feelings without fear of being misunderstood or minimized.

Secondly, emotional support must aim to **alleviate the anxieties** associated with the disease and its treatment. Patients may feel existential anxiety about the chronicity of their pathology, fearing that they will never regain their previous quality of life, or that they will be a burden to their loved ones. Caregivers can play a calming role by explaining the course of treatment, patiently answering questions and offering constant emotional support. It is also helpful to encourage patients to remain active and involved in their own treatment, which can give them back a sense of control and reduce their anxiety.

Emotional support is not just about listening or calming fears; it also includes encouragement to maintain optimism and **boost self-esteem**. Kidney disease can profoundly affect a patient's self-perception, due to chronic fatigue, dietary restrictions, or the physical limitations imposed by treatment. It's important to recognize these difficulties while emphasizing the positive aspects, valuing the efforts the patient makes to manage his disease, and encouraging him to maintain even modest goals in his day-to-day life.

Caregivers can also accompany patients in **activities that promote their emotional well-being**, whether these involve social activities, adapted leisure activities, or moments of relaxation. Proposing solutions such as meditation, guided relaxation, or even group discussions with other patients can help relieve stress and create a sense of solidarity, reducing the isolation often felt in the care process.

Balancing ethics and emotions: comprehensive patient care

Ethical and emotional support must work in complementary ways. While ethical support ensures that the patient's choices, values and rights are respected, emotional support enables them to find human support, to feel understood and accompanied in their care journey. By combining these two dimensions, the caregiver ensures that not only the patient's illness is treated, but also the whole person, taking into account his or her physical, mental and spiritual needs.

This balance is particularly important at critical moments, such as the end of life or the cessation of heavy treatment. Patients, and often their families, may need both ethical support, to help them make difficult decisions while respecting their wishes, and emotional support, to help them cope with the psychological upheaval these decisions entail. Careful, attentive support can help them to get through these difficult times with greater serenity, while offering them a dignified end-of-life experience in keeping with their own values.

Chapter 8

The specificities of care for kidney transplant patients

- **Understanding kidney transplantation**: the stages of transplantation and post-operative follow-up.

Kidney transplantation is often the preferred treatment option for patients with end-stage renal disease, as it can offer a better quality of life and greater autonomy than dialysis. However, the kidney transplant process is complex, requiring careful preparation, delicate surgery and rigorous post-operative follow-up to ensure long-term success. Understanding the different stages of this process, from initial assessment through to post-transplant follow-up, provides a better understanding of the challenges and care required for the patient.

Stages of renal transplantation: from evaluation to transplantation

The first step before a kidney transplant is to **assess the patient** to make sure he or she is a suitable candidate. This assessment is multidisciplinary and includes thorough medical examinations, blood tests, imaging tests, and consultations with various specialists. The aim is to verify that the patient is healthy enough to undergo transplantation and to withstand long-term immunosuppressive treatments. We must also ensure that the patient has no major contraindications, such as active infections, severe cardiovascular disease or uncontrolled cancer.

Alongside the medical assessment, there is often a **psychological and social evaluation** to ensure that the patient is ready to manage the demands of a transplant and post-operative follow-up. It is essential to check that the patient fully understands the implications of the transplant, including scrupulous adherence to immunosuppressive treatment and regular consultations. Family and social support also play an important role in this phase, as the patient will need a stable environment for convalescence.

Once the assessment has been completed and validated, the patient is placed on the **transplant waiting list**, unless he or she is a living donor. In the case of deceased donor transplants, waiting times can vary considerably, depending on organ compatibility and availability. Compatibility is determined by immunological criteria, such as blood group compatibility and tissue compatibility tests (HLA). When a compatible kidney is available, the patient is urgently contacted to go to hospital for the transplant.

The **transplant surgery** itself involves implanting the donor kidney into the patient's lower abdomen, without removing the failing kidneys, except in cases of complications (such as chronic infection). The artery and vein of the transplanted kidney are connected to the recipient's blood vessels, and the ureter of the new kidney is connected to the bladder to enable urine elimination. Surgery generally lasts between three and four hours and is performed under general anaesthetic.

Immediate post-operative care: the critical first few days

The days following the kidney transplant are critical, as the body must adapt to the transplanted organ and begin to function with the new kidney. The patient is placed under **intensive surveillance** for the first 48 to 72 hours to ensure that the transplanted kidney begins to produce urine and that vital signs are stable. Frequent blood tests ensure that the kidney is functioning properly, by monitoring markers such as creatinine and electrolytes. Good urine production in the hours following transplant is generally a positive sign of kidney function.

However, during this critical phase, the risk of **acute rejection** is high. Acute rejection occurs when the patient's immune system recognizes the transplanted kidney as a foreign body and attempts to attack it. To prevent this reaction, **immunosuppressive drugs** are administered immediately after transplantation. These drugs weaken the immune system so that it does not reject the transplanted organ. Immunosuppressive treatment is intensive for the first few days, requiring precise adjustment of doses according to the patient's response. Biopsies of the transplanted kidney may be taken if rejection is suspected, in order to adapt the treatment.

In addition to rejection, other post-operative complications can arise, such as infections, blood clots and scarring problems. This is why the patient remains hospitalized for several days, or even weeks, for close monitoring. The medical team also checks the kidney for vascular problems, such as renal artery stenosis, which could compromise its proper functioning.

Long-term follow-up: preventing rejection and managing immunosuppressants

Once the immediate post-operative period is over, long-term follow-up begins, and this is a crucial phase in guaranteeing graft survival. The patient must take **immunosuppressive drugs for life**, because even after several months or years, the risk of chronic rejection persists. Treatment generally involves a combination of several drugs, such as cyclosporine, tacrolimus or mycophenolate mofetil, which act by blocking different immune system pathways.

Medical follow-up includes regular consultations with the nephrologist, **frequent blood tests** to monitor kidney function, and examinations to check the levels of immunosuppressive drugs in the blood. These checks are essential because too low a dosage of immunosuppressants can lead to rejection, while too high a dosage exposes the patient to infections or serious side effects, such as liver problems or kidney toxicity.

Transplant patients are particularly vulnerable to **infection**, due to immunosuppression, which weakens their ability to fight pathogens. They must therefore be extremely vigilant when it comes to hygiene, and avoid all contact with people with viral or bacterial infections. Specific vaccinations may be recommended, but only with inactivated vaccines, as live attenuated vaccines can be dangerous for patients on immunosuppressive therapy.

The risk of **chronic rejection** is a constant concern, even several years after transplantation. This type of rejection occurs more slowly and can lead to a progressive deterioration in kidney function. Regular biopsies may be necessary to detect the first signs of chronic rejection and adapt treatment. It is important that the patient adhere strictly to the immunosuppressive treatment, without missing doses, and that he/she consults immediately in the event of symptoms such as reduced urine production, abnormal fatigue, or pain at the graft site.

Quality of life after transplant: regaining a sense of normalcy

For many patients, a kidney transplant represents a veritable renaissance after years of dialysis or suffering from kidney failure. Although daily immunosuppressive therapy and regular consultations remain a lifelong necessity, transplantation often enables patients to regain greater freedom, a better quality of life, and a much better general state of health than on dialysis.

Transplant patients can generally resume a more active lifestyle, with fewer dietary restrictions and better hydration management. However, it is crucial that they continue to follow certain recommendations to preserve their graft, such as avoiding situations at risk of infection, watching their weight, controlling their blood pressure, and adopting a healthy lifestyle.

For many, transplantation enables them to return to work, physical activity and normal social interaction, giving them the independence that dialysis no longer afforded. However, the long-term success of transplantation depends on rigorous adherence to treatment and medical follow-up, and careful risk management.

- **Post-transplant patient management**: monitoring for signs of rejection, management of immunosuppressive treatments.

Monitoring for signs of rejection and managing immunosuppressive therapy are two essential pillars in the follow-up of transplant patients, particularly after kidney transplantation. After transplantation, the patient's immune system, even when weakened by immunosuppressants, may identify the new kidney as a foreign body and attempt to attack it, leading to organ rejection. Careful monitoring of kidney function and rigorous management of immunosuppressive drugs are therefore crucial to preventing and treating such rejection, thus prolonging graft life and ensuring patient stability.

Monitoring signs of rejection: identifying early symptoms

Graft rejection can occur at different times, either shortly after transplantation (acute rejection), or months or years later (chronic rejection). Each type of rejection has its own characteristics, but it's essential that the patient and the health-care team are vigilant in recognizing the early signs of rejection, so they can intervene quickly.

In the case of **acute rejection**, which generally occurs in the first days or weeks following transplantation, symptoms can be sudden and severe. The patient may experience decreased urine production, pain or tenderness at the graft site, unexplained fever, rapid weight gain due to fluid retention, or extreme fatigue. Blood tests often reveal a rapid rise in creatinine, which is a direct indicator of reduced renal function. Acute rejection, if detected in time, can often be treated with higher doses of immunosuppressants, or by the addition of specific drugs to modulate the immune response.

Chronic rejection, on the other hand, is more insidious. It develops slowly and can sometimes go unnoticed for several months. This type of rejection manifests itself through a progressive deterioration in renal function, often revealed by a slow but steady rise in creatinine levels in blood tests, as well as general symptoms such as fatigue, hypertension and reduced urine production. Unlike acute rejection, chronic rejection is more difficult to treat, as it corresponds to a prolonged and subtle immune reaction that causes permanent damage to the transplanted kidney tissue.

Patients must be educated from the outset to recognize these symptoms and know when to alert their doctor. It's important never to overlook abnormal fatigue, altered diuresis, or rapid weight gain, even if these symptoms may seem harmless. **Regular monitoring of blood** tests can detect abnormalities before they become clinically apparent. In case of doubt, further tests, such as a graft biopsy, may be carried out to confirm the diagnosis of rejection.

Managing immunosuppressive treatments: a delicate balance

Immunosuppressive therapy is essential to prevent graft rejection, but requires meticulous management as these drugs have powerful effects on the immune system and can lead to significant complications. The aim of immunosuppressants is to reduce immune system activity sufficiently to prevent kidney rejection without exposing the patient to an increased risk of infection or cancer. Striking this balance is often a challenge for doctors, and requires careful monitoring.

The treatment regimen for **immunosuppressants** generally includes several classes of drugs that act on different parts of the immune system. Patients often take a combination of drugs such as cyclosporine, tacrolimus, mycophenolate mofetil or corticosteroids. These drugs are generally administered for life, and dosage must be adjusted regularly according to changes in renal function, side effects and blood test results.

The **dosage of immunosuppressants** is extremely precise and must be closely monitored to avoid two opposing scenarios: under-immunosuppression, which can lead to graft rejection, or over-immunosuppression, which exposes the patient to serious infections or other complications, such as kidney or liver toxicity. Blood levels of drugs such as cyclosporine or tacrolimus are measured regularly to ensure that they are within a safe therapeutic range.

One of the most frequent consequences of immunosuppression is an **increased risk of infection**, as the immune system is weakened. Transplant patients must be particularly vigilant and adopt strict hygiene measures to avoid exposure to pathogens. Viral, bacterial or fungal infections can rapidly become serious in these patients, necessitating hospitalization or treatment adjustments. Vaccinations (excluding live attenuated vaccines) are generally recommended to boost protection against certain infections, but the decision to vaccinate will depend on the patient's condition and the medications he or she is taking.

In addition to infections, immunosuppressants can have other **long-term side effects**, such as osteoporosis, hypertension, diabetes and skin cancer. Patients must therefore be regularly monitored by their medical team to detect these complications as early as possible. For example, regular dermatological examinations are necessary to monitor the occurrence of skin cancers, and preventive measures such as the use of sunscreens should be encouraged.

The importance of treatment adherence: avoiding interruptions

One of the keys to long-term transplant success is **adherence to immunosuppressive therapy**. Patients need to understand that even an oversight or delay in taking their medication can put their graft at risk. Unlike other treatments, immunosuppressants require strict regularity. Failure to do so can rapidly lead to acute rejection, with potentially irreversible consequences.

It is therefore crucial to **make patients aware** of the importance of taking their medication regularly, by providing them with practical tools such as pillboxes or telephone reminders so they don't forget their doses. The healthcare team also needs to establish an open dialogue with the patient to understand any difficulties he or she may have in following the treatment, and propose appropriate solutions. For example, if a patient experiences troublesome effects-side, it is essential to discuss them with the doctor to adjust the treatment rather than risk stopping the medication.

- **The role of the caregiver in rehabilitation and reintegration**: Encouraging mobility and daily activities.

Encouraging mobility and daily activities is a key element in the care of kidney disease patients, whether on dialysis or transplant. Maintaining an appropriate level of physical activity and encouraging autonomy in daily activities have considerable physical and psychological benefits. Mobility helps prevent complications associated with prolonged immobility, while daily activities help maintain dignity and self-esteem. In this context, the caregiver plays a crucial role in accompanying the patient towards greater autonomy, while ensuring that advice and exercises are adapted to each individual's abilities and state of health.

Importance of mobility: preventing physical complications

Even reduced mobility is essential to avoid the complications associated with prolonged immobilization. Patients on dialysis or in end-stage renal failure can quickly feel tired, which often leads them to remain inactive. However, this inactivity can lead to a deterioration in general condition, with increased risks of muscle loss, osteoporosis, respiratory disorders and cardiovascular complications. Encouraging mobility helps counteract these effects, and improves blood circulation, breathing and muscle tone.

For kidney failure patients, regular exercise helps to keep joints supple and prevent mobility problems. Gentle exercises, such as walking, stretching, or adapted activities, can be encouraged according to the patient's abilities. The aim is not to impose an intensive exercise program, but to promote **regular physical activity**, even in moderation, which contributes to maintaining good general health.

For dialysis patients, mobility is just as crucial. Dialysis can cause periods of intense fatigue, but remaining inactive during and after dialysis can lead to complications such as muscle cramps, edema or low morale. Encouraging patients to get up and walk as soon as possible after dialysis, or even to perform simple movements during the session (such as light leg or arm exercises), can help improve tolerance to treatment and prevent muscle atrophy.

Reintegrating daily activities: regaining independence

In addition to mobility, the **reintegration of daily activities** into the patient's routine is essential for his or her autonomy and well-being. Even mundane activities such as washing, dressing, preparing meals or moving around the home have a direct impact on self-esteem. Being able to perform these tasks without assistance enhances the patient's dignity and enables him or her to regain a sense of control over his or her body and life.

For transplant patients or those in the advanced stages of the disease, it can be difficult to regain this autonomy quickly, due to fatigue, physical restrictions or pain. That's why it's important to **support** them **gradually** in reintegrating daily activities, starting with small tasks and gradually increasing the level of complexity according to their abilities. For example, a patient recovering from a kidney transplant may start by moving around their room, then gradually be encouraged to prepare a simple meal or take a short walk outside.

Caregivers must be vigilant, adapting their support to the patient's abilities. It is important not to force patients to go beyond what they can do, but rather to encourage them to maintain their independence by helping them find solutions to overcome their difficulties. This can include **practical adjustments** to the environment, such as the use of shower chairs, support bars or ergonomic equipment to facilitate certain gestures.

Beneficial effects on mental health and quality of life

Encouraging mobility and engagement in daily activities also has a positive impact on patients' mental health. Kidney disease, particularly when it requires dialysis or transplantation, is often experienced as a loss of control over one's body and life. This feeling of powerlessness can lead to anxiety, depression and stress. Being able to resume simple everyday activities, or to move around even in a modest way, can **boost self-confidence** and bring positive structure to a patient's day.

Active mobility and daily activities promote the production of endorphins, wellness hormones that help improve mood and reduce feelings of fatigue or pain. This is particularly important for transplant patients, who often have to adapt to a new post-transplant reality, and for dialysis patients, who may feel physically and mentally exhausted by the pace of sessions.

What's more, being **active** helps to **break down isolation**. A patient who manages to get out of the house, even for a short walk or to visit friends, will be more inclined to maintain social interactions and stay involved in daily life. Support from caregivers, but also from loved ones, can play a crucial role in this dynamic. Offering activities adapted to the patient's abilities, such as outings to parks or light group activities, can reinforce social integration and promote a better quality of life.

Personalized guidance and moral support

Encouragement of mobility and daily activities must be tailored to each individual patient. Not all patients react in the same way to illness, and some may feel more fragile than others. Support must therefore be **adapted** to each patient's **physical capabilities**, emotional state and individual preferences.

For example, a dialysis patient may prefer gentle exercise, such as light stretching or outdoor walks, while a transplant patient in the recovery phase may be encouraged to gradually resume his or her domestic and social habits. It's important to respect the patient's pace, while offering constant moral support to encourage him or her to keep progressing, even in the face of obstacles or periods of fatigue.

Moral support is also essential in this process. For some patients, reintegration into daily activities may seem difficult or discouraging. In such cases, the caregiver plays a key role in valuing each small step forward, offering encouragement and emphasizing the long-term benefits of mobility. It's also crucial to understand the psychological disincentives some patients may feel, such as fear of pain or failure, and to help them overcome these fears by adopting a progressive, caring approach.

Chapter 9

Prevention and therapeutic education in nephrology

- **The importance of therapeutic education**: Helping patients understand their disease.

Helping patients to understand their illness is an essential task in the management of kidney disease, whether they suffer from chronic renal failure, are on dialysis, or are waiting for a transplant. A good understanding of the disease helps patients to accept their situation, adapt their lifestyle and adhere more easily to treatment. As a caregiver, explaining the pathology in clear, accessible terms that are adapted to each patient helps them to take charge of their own health. This helps to reduce the anxiety associated with uncertainty and feelings of powerlessness, by helping patients to regain control over certain aspects of their daily lives.

Explain the disease in a simple and appropriate way

The first step in helping patients understand their disease is to provide clear explanations adapted to their level of understanding. Kidney disease, particularly chronic renal failure, can seem complex and frightening, especially to someone with no medical background. It is therefore crucial to translate technical terms into simple language, without infantilizing or downplaying the seriousness of the situation.

For example, to explain how the kidneys work and how they fail, it may be useful to compare the kidneys to **natural filters** that clean the blood by removing waste and excess water. When these filters no longer function properly, waste accumulates in the body, which can make a person ill. This type of metaphor helps patients visualize what's going on in their bodies and understand why they experience certain symptoms, such as fatigue, edema or high blood pressure.

It's also important to explain the **stage of the disease**. Chronic renal failure generally develops in stages, from mild impairment of kidney function to complete failure requiring dialysis or transplantation. By explaining where the patient is in this journey, we can give them a clearer picture of their current situation and

114

what they can expect. It also enables clear goals to be set, such as slowing disease progression through lifestyle changes or anticipating future treatments.

Clarify treatments and their objectives

Once the disease has been explained, it's essential to talk about treatments in a detailed and accessible way. For a patient, treatments such as dialysis, transplants or immunosuppressants can seem daunting. The key to helping them understand and accept these treatments is to **break down each aspect of** the treatment, explaining why it's necessary, how it works, and what the long-term benefits are.

In the case of dialysis, for example, explaining that the process replaces the kidneys' filtration function by cleansing the blood helps explain why sessions are necessary several times a week. It's also important to discuss **possible side effects** (fatigue, low blood pressure, cramps) and how to manage them. The information given should not be purely theoretical, but should include practical advice to help patients live better with their treatment.

If the patient is waiting for or has received a transplant, it is also important to explain what **immunosuppressive treatments** are, why they must be taken for life, and what risks are associated with poor compliance. This explanation should be accompanied by advice on how to manage the treatments on a daily basis, such as the use of reminders so as not to forget to take the medication.

Encourage interaction and answer questions

A patient who understands his or her illness is one who feels free to ask questions. Encouraging patients to **actively participate** in discussions about their health is essential to improving their understanding. This can be done by creating a climate of trust, explaining that all questions, even the simplest or those that seem repetitive, are important.

It's also useful to regularly rephrase what the patient has understood, by asking, for example, "Can you tell me in your own words what you've retained about your treatment?" or "What worries you most about your illness?" These questions help to identify areas of misunderstanding and remedy them before they become obstacles to treatment adherence.

What's more, every patient is unique and experiences his or her illness in a different way. Some patients may need more time to assimilate information, while others may feel overwhelmed by the mass of medical details. Adapting the frequency and pace of explanations to suit the patient's needs and anxiety level helps ensure that they don't feel rushed or abandoned. Offering visual or written aids, such as brochures or diagrams, can also reinforce understanding by giving patients a point of reference they can consult at any time.

Provide psychological and emotional support

Understanding your illness goes beyond simply explaining the medical facts. It also involves the **emotional acceptance of** pathology. Chronic kidney disease, for example, is an irreversible condition that profoundly changes a patient's life. It is therefore essential not to neglect the psychological aspect of this support.

Some patients may feel angry, anxious or discouraged by the progression of their disease or the burdensome nature of their treatment. Explaining the disease with kindness and empathy can help them overcome these emotions. By acknowledging that illness can be a difficult experience, the caregiver validates the patient's feelings and shows them that they are not alone in this process. This emotional validation is just as important as medical explanations, helping to reduce stress and facilitate acceptance of the situation.

Another aspect of emotional support is reminding patients that they can **play an active role** in managing their disease. This can be done by giving them practical advice on how to take care of themselves on a daily basis, such as following a suitable diet, monitoring their fluid intake, or incorporating gentle physical activity into their routine. This kind of advice empowers the patient and makes him feel less helpless in the face of his illness.

Strengthening treatment adherence through understanding

One of the main benefits of helping patients understand their disease is to improve their **adherence to treatment**. A patient who understands why they need to follow a certain prescription is more likely to stick to it over the long term. This is particularly important in chronic diseases such as renal failure, where failure to follow recommendations can have serious consequences, such as worsening the disease or graft failure.

Adherence to treatment can be reinforced by regular discussion of disease progression and test results. For example, explaining to patients how creatinine and electrolyte monitoring can measure the effectiveness of their treatment or prevent complications encourages them to follow their check-ups closely. Similarly, stressing the importance of regular medical appointments to adjust medication doses or monitor for any signs of rejection helps patients better understand the role of each stage in their care.

- **The caregiver's role in preventing complications**: advice on healthy living and regular monitoring.

Lifestyle advice and regular monitoring are essential pillars in the management of patients with kidney disease, whether on dialysis, transplant or chronic renal failure. An adapted lifestyle, coupled with rigorous medical monitoring, not only slows disease progression, but also improves quality of life and prevents complications. These recommendations, which cover diet, physical activity, stress management and compliance with medical consultations, help patients to take an active role in managing their disease.

Adopting the right diet: a key to healthy living

Diet plays a crucial role in the management of kidney disease, as damaged kidneys can no longer effectively eliminate certain excess minerals or toxins from the blood. Diet must therefore be strictly controlled and adapted to the patient's needs, depending on the stage of the disease, treatment (dialysis or transplant) and general condition.

A **low-sodium** diet is one of the first recommendations. Reducing salt in the diet helps prevent hypertension and water retention, two frequent complications in kidney patients. This means avoiding processed foods rich in salt, such as ready-made meals, cold meats and preserves, and favoring fresh ingredients, using herbs and spices to enhance the taste of dishes without adding salt.

Reducing **potassium** intake is also crucial, especially for patients on dialysis. Diseased kidneys can no longer effectively eliminate excess potassium, which can lead to potentially serious heart rhythm disorders. Patients should therefore limit potassium-rich foods such as bananas, potatoes, tomatoes and dried fruit. Dietary advice can include food preparation methods, such as boiling vegetables to reduce their potassium content.

Phosphorus is another mineral to watch out for, as phosphorus build-up in the blood can lead to bone and cardiovascular problems. Limiting dairy products, legumes and certain meats rich in phosphorus is often necessary, while ensuring that these restrictions are offset by adequate protein intakes, according to the patient's individual needs.

Personalized dietary support is essential to adjust these recommendations to the specific preferences and needs of each patient, while ensuring that they maintain a balanced and pleasant diet.

Maintaining appropriate physical activity: preserving physical and mental well-being

Physical activity is another fundamental aspect of a healthy lifestyle for kidney disease patients. It not only helps prevent muscle atrophy and weight gain, but also reduces hypertension, promotes better blood sugar management, and improves morale. It is important to adapt the intensity of physical activity to the patient's state of health, as some patients may quickly feel tired or suffer from pain.

Recommended exercises are often **moderate** but regular, such as walking, gentle cycling or stretching. For dialysis patients, light exercises can be performed between or even during dialysis sessions to maintain blood circulation and prevent muscle cramps. The aim is to maintain flexibility and improve physical condition without overtaxing a body already weakened by the disease.

Physical activity also has **psychological benefits**. It releases endorphins, hormones that promote a sense of well-being and relaxation, reducing the symptoms of stress and depression often associated with chronic illness. Encouraging regular exercise, even in moderation, helps patients to feel more in control of their health and improve their self-esteem.

Managing stress and taking care of your mental health

Stress management is an often underestimated but crucial aspect in the lifestyle of kidney disease patients. The progression of the disease, heavy treatments such as dialysis, and uncertainty about the future often generate anxiety and mental fatigue. Learning to manage these emotions is essential to avoid psychological exhaustion and maintain a good quality of life.

Relaxation techniques such as meditation, deep breathing or gentle yoga can help reduce stress and improve concentration.

These practices promote better emotional management and can be easily integrated into patients' daily routines. For those who feel particularly anxious, psychological support, through individual or group therapy, can also be very beneficial.

Social support also plays a key role in stress management. Patients with kidney disease can sometimes feel isolated because of their illness, which can exacerbate anxiety and depression. It's important for them to be able to count on their loved ones, but also on support networks, such as patient groups, to share their experiences and feel less alone in their care journey.

Regular medical check-ups: an essential element in preventing complications

Regular medical follow-up is undoubtedly one of the most important factors in ensuring optimal care for patients with kidney disease. It enables us to monitor the evolution of kidney function, adjust treatments according to the results of check-ups, and prevent complications linked to the disease or the treatments themselves.

Regular blood tests are essential for monitoring key parameters such as creatinine, urea, potassium and phosphorus, as well as for checking drug levels, especially for patients on dialysis or immunosuppressive therapy after transplantation. These analyses enable early detection of any abnormalities and adjustment of treatments before serious symptoms appear.

In transplant patients, regular consultations monitor signs of **graft rejection** and ensure that immunosuppressive treatments are well balanced. Close monitoring also enables early detection of side effects, such as infections or skin cancer, and preventive or corrective action.

It is also crucial to **educate patients** on the importance of keeping medical appointments and not interrupting or modifying their treatment without medical advice. Some patients may underestimate the importance of regular check-ups, especially when they're feeling well, but it's vital to remind them that kidney disease, even when stabilized, requires constant vigilance.

- **Working with patients and their families**: Supporting and training caregivers.

Supporting and training caregivers is an essential part of caring for patients with chronic kidney disease or end-stage renal failure. Caregivers, whether family members or close friends, play a key role in patients' daily lives, providing physical, emotional and often medical support. They help manage day-to-day tasks, monitor treatment compliance, and offer moral support in the face of the challenges posed by the disease. However, this role can be challenging, both physically and psychologically, and it is essential that caregivers are trained and supported to better understand the disease, its treatments and their implications.

Understanding the central role of caregivers

Caregivers are often the link between the patient and the medical team. They help arrange medical appointments, monitor symptoms, make sure the patient is following his or her treatment, and intervene in emergencies. However, without proper training and support, this burden can quickly become onerous. It is therefore crucial to recognize the importance of their role and integrate them fully into the care process.

One of the first steps in supporting caregivers is to **provide** them **with the necessary information** on kidney disease and treatment. This involves explaining in simple but precise terms how the kidneys work, the progression of kidney failure, and the impact of treatments such as dialysis or transplantation. Basic training enables them to better understand what the patient is going through, and how to react to unforeseen situations. In addition, providing them with resources on symptom management - such as observing signs of graft rejection or monitoring dialysis-related complications - helps them to make informed decisions on a daily basis.

Training caregivers in technical gestures

In some cases, caregivers are required to perform technical tasks, such as monitoring blood pressure, managing home dialysis equipment or administering certain medications. It is therefore essential to train them in these practices in a clear and practical way, with concrete demonstrations and detailed explanations. For example, a caregiver can be trained to manage home peritoneal dialysis, which involves preparing sterile equipment, monitoring complications such as infections, and ensuring that the patient complies with schedules and instructions.

Caregivers also need to learn how to **react in the event of an emergency**, be it patient discomfort, severe hypotension during dialysis, or the first signs of acute rejection after a transplant. Providing them with clear and simple action protocols to follow in these situations helps to reassure them and reinforce their effectiveness. Regular training and review sessions can also be offered to keep their skills up to date, and enable them to ask questions when in doubt.

Emotional support for caregivers

Beyond the technical aspects, emotional support for caregivers is just as crucial. Caring for a sick loved one can be psychologically exhausting, especially when the illness is chronic and progressive. Caregivers are often faced with a mixture of stress, fatigue and guilt, due to feelings of not doing enough or of being helpless in the face of the patient's suffering. This emotional burden, if left unchecked, can lead to **psychological exhaustion** or a deterioration in their own health.

It is therefore essential to **listen to caregivers**, to recognize their difficulties, and to offer them a forum where they can express their fears, frustrations and doubts without being judged. Carers can encourage caregivers to join support groups or patient associations, where they can talk to others in similar situations. These exchanges help to break down isolation, share practical tips, and find moral support from people who fully understand the challenges they face.

Preventing caregiver burnout

Caregiver exhaustion, often referred to as "caregiver burn-out", is a real risk when caregivers are overburdened, without respite or adequate support. Caring for a sick loved one while managing their own responsibilities (work, family, etc.) can lead to physical and emotional exhaustion, damaging their well-being and their ability to help the patient effectively.

It's crucial to remind caregivers that it's essential to **take care of themselves** so they can continue to help their loved ones. This means taking time out for rest and personal activities, and sometimes using home help or respite services to take over temporarily. Caregivers can also point them in the direction of practical solutions, such as financial aid, support services or logistical solutions to lighten their daily burden.

Time management is another key aspect. It is useful to provide caregivers with advice on care planning, so that they can organize their days in a balanced way, including moments of pause for themselves. Delegating certain tasks to other family members or healthcare professionals can also be considered, to avoid one caregiver carrying the whole load.

Involving caregivers in medical decisions

One of the most effective ways of supporting caregivers is to **involve** them **fully in medical decisions concerning** the patient. By informing them of the various treatment options and decisions to be made, they feel less helpless in the face of the disease and can play an active role in its management. They will be better prepared to support the patient and help him or her make informed decisions.

This involvement in medical discussions also reinforces their sense of belonging to the healthcare team, and helps them better understand the issues involved in treatment and care. This reduces their anxiety and gives them the tools they need to support the patient in a more informed and confident way.

Chapter 10

Emergency management in nephrology

- **Renal emergencies: hyperkalemia, pulmonary edema, hypovolemic shock**: how to recognize and respond.

Renal emergencies, such as hyperkalemia, pulmonary edema and hypovolemic shock, represent critical situations that can arise in patients suffering from renal failure or on dialysis. These conditions require rapid, effective intervention to prevent serious, even life-threatening complications. Recognizing early clinical signs and knowing how to respond to them is essential to ensure the patient's survival and well-being. These emergencies often involve metabolic and fluid imbalances, aggravated by the failure of the kidneys to maintain an adequate internal balance.

Hyperkalemia: an electrolyte imbalance that threatens the heart

Hyperkalemia is an excessive elevation of potassium in the blood, and is common in patients with chronic renal failure, as their kidneys are no longer able to eliminate this mineral properly. Potassium plays a vital role in regulating muscular contractions, particularly those of the heart. Untreated hyperkalemia can lead to **serious heart rhythm disorders** and even cardiac arrest.

The clinical signs of hyperkalemia are often subtle at first, but can quickly become threatening. Symptoms include **muscle weakness**, **palpitations**, **tingling** or numbness in the extremities, and impaired consciousness in advanced cases. At a more critical stage, **electrocardiographic (ECG) changes** appear, with T-wave peaks, widening of the QRS complex, and possibly asystole.

When hyperkalemia is suspected, an **immediate blood test** is required to confirm the diagnosis by measuring potassium levels. Treatment of hyperkalemia aims to stabilize the heart and rapidly reduce potassium levels. A first line of defense is to administer **intravenous calcium** to protect the heart from the toxic effects of potassium. Simultaneously, treatments to lower potassium levels can be administered, such as glucose-coupled insulin, which helps move potassium into the cells, or beta-agonists.

In cases of severe or persistent hyperkalemia, **emergency dialysis** may be required to rapidly remove potassium from the blood. Prevention of hyperkalemia involves regular monitoring of electrolytes, adjustment of diet (including reduction of potassium-rich foods), and adherence to diuretic therapy or dialysis for patients concerned.

Pulmonary edema: acute fluid overload

Pulmonary edema is a sudden accumulation of fluid in the lungs, often caused by **fluid overload** in patients with renal failure. The failing kidneys cannot properly eliminate excess fluid, leading to increased pressure in the pulmonary vessels, causing fluid to flood the pulmonary alveoli. This prevents proper oxygenation of the blood and can rapidly become fatal if not promptly treated.

Clinical signs of acute pulmonary oedema include **sudden respiratory distress**, with a sensation of shortness of air (dyspnoea), **rapid**, shallow **breathing**, a **productive cough** with frothy, sometimes blood-tinged sputum, and a **crackling rattle** heard on auscultation of the lungs. In severe cases, the patient's skin may become **cold and clammy**, and signs of cyanosis (bluish coloration of the lips and extremities) may appear, indicating insufficient oxygenation of the blood.

Management of acute pulmonary edema must be immediate. The first step is to **administer oxygen** to improve oxygenation and relieve respiratory distress. In severe cases, intubation and mechanical ventilation may be necessary. Treatment aims to reduce fluid overload by administering **potent diuretics** (such as furosemide), which help to eliminate excess fluid rapidly. In some cases, emergency dialysis may be required to remove excess fluid when the kidneys are no longer able to do so.

Prevention of pulmonary edema relies on **strict control of fluid intake** and regular monitoring of weight and signs of fluid accumulation (peripheral edema, rapid weight gain). Adjustment of diuretic doses or more frequent management of dialysis sessions may be necessary to avoid episodes of fluid overload.

Hypovolemic shock: a sudden loss of blood volume

Hypovolemic shock is a life-threatening emergency that occurs when a significant loss of fluid or blood causes a sudden drop in the body's circulating volume, compromising the heart's ability to pump blood efficiently to the organs. In patients with renal failure or on dialysis, hypovolemic shock can be caused by severe dehydration (due to excessive dialysis or poorly managed fluid intake), significant blood loss during surgery or digestive bleeding.

Symptoms of hypovolemic shock are usually rapid and include **severe hypotension**, **compensatory tachycardia** (rapid increase in heart rate), **pallor** and **cold extremities**, **intense thirst**, **confusion** or loss of consciousness in the most severe cases. At this stage, the vital organs no longer receive sufficient blood, and multivisceral failure can occur if shock is not treated quickly.

Management of hypovolemic shock requires **immediate volume resuscitation**. This involves rapid intravenous administration of crystalloid solutions to restore circulating blood volume. In cases of hemorrhagic shock, **blood transfusions** may be necessary to replace lost blood. At the same time, it is crucial to **identify and treat the underlying cause of** the shock, whether it be hemorrhage or severe dehydration.

Treatment of hypovolemic shock is a race against time to restore perfusion to vital organs. Continuous monitoring of blood pressure, heart rate and diuresis is necessary to assess treatment efficacy. Prevention of this condition requires **rigorous management of fluid and blood intake** in patients at risk, as well as increased vigilance in the post-operative period or during dialysis sessions, when fluid imbalances may occur.

- **The caregiver's first response to a patient's deteriorating condition**: Reflexes to have before the nurse or doctor intervenes.

When caring for patients with kidney disease or undergoing dialysis treatment, it's crucial that caregivers, orderlies and even relatives have the right reflexes before a nurse or doctor intervenes. These emergency or distress situations can be moments of great confusion and panic. Knowing how to act quickly and effectively before medical professionals arrive can make a significant difference to the patient's condition. This involves not only recognizing the warning signs of a problem, but also knowing what immediate action to take to stabilize the situation.

Observing and assessing the situation: a crucial first step

The first thing to do is to **calmly observe** and **assess** the situation. Understanding what is happening is essential to determining the urgency of the situation. This means paying attention to the patient's vital signs and general condition: level of consciousness, breathing, skin color, behavior and response to stimuli. Is he conscious? Is he breathing normally? Is he agitated, confused or apathetic? These are invaluable clues for directing the first steps.

It's important to **remain calm** so as not to aggravate the situation, as a panicked reaction can lead to mistakes or poor choices. Careful observation can help identify signs of seriousness, such as difficulty breathing (dyspnea), sudden confusion, intense pain or loss of consciousness. Once this information has been collected, it must be quickly communicated to the nurse or doctor, to enable them to better apprehend the situation on arrival.

Position the patient correctly: immediate relief

While waiting for help to arrive, the **patient's position** can sometimes improve comfort or even prevent a deterioration in his or her condition. In the event of breathing difficulties, as in pulmonary edema, it is advisable to place the patient in a **semi-seated position**, with support for the back, to facilitate breathing. This helps to reduce pressure on the lungs and improve oxygenation while waiting for a more specific intervention.

In the event of discomfort with a drop in blood pressure, it may be helpful to **place the patient in a supine position with legs elevated** (decubitus dorsi). This position, known as the modified Trendelenburg position, helps to promote venous return and stabilize blood pressure. If the patient is showing signs of shock or severe hypotension, this position can prevent symptoms from worsening before caregivers arrive.

It's also important to keep patients **warm**, especially if they show signs of shock, such as cold, clammy skin. Using blankets or extra clothing can help prevent hypothermia, especially in situations of cardiac or vascular distress.

Check and stabilize vital signs: breathing and circulation

In the event of respiratory distress, **vital signs** must be carefully monitored. Observation of respiratory rate, oxygen saturation (if a pulse oximeter is available), and heart rate can give important clues to the severity of the situation. If the patient has difficulty breathing, an oxygen mask can be applied if the equipment is available, or simple measures such as opening windows to bring in fresh air can help improve oxygenation.

If the patient shows signs of **hypovolemic shock** or hypotension (extreme weakness, pale skin, rapid and weak pulse), it is important to monitor pulse and blood pressure. While waiting for the nurse or doctor to intervene, these parameters should continue to be monitored regularly, and any changes noted, so as to provide clear information to caregivers when they arrive.

Helping manage hyperkalemia: act quickly if signs appear

In the event that a patient with renal failure shows signs suggestive of hyperkalemia, such as palpitations, muscle weakness or sudden fatigue, it is imperative to **react quickly**. Although specific treatment must await the intervention of a physician, certain measures can be taken to temporarily stabilize the patient. For example, avoiding physical exertion can reduce the risk of cardiac complications by slowing down muscle and heart activity.

It is also important to avoid **sources of potassium** in the diet if the patient is conscious and able to eat. In the absence of immediate treatment, this can limit a worsening of the situation.

Reassuring the patient: psychological and verbal support

In emergency situations, patient anxiety can worsen their condition, particularly in cases of respiratory distress or intense pain. One of the essential reflexes before medical staff intervene is to **reassure the patient**. Talking to them gently, calmly explaining what's happening, and assuring them that help is on the way can reduce their anxiety and help prevent a panic attack that could complicate the situation.

This psychological support is essential, as anxiety can accelerate breathing (tachypnea) and worsen a situation of respiratory or cardiovascular distress. Simple gestures such as holding the patient's hand, asking them to breathe slowly and deeply, or reminding them that they are not alone can have an immediate calming effect.

Assessing and stopping sources of risk: safety and the environment

If the emergency has arisen from a specific incident, such as a fall or injury, it is important to **eliminate** immediate **sources of danger** before the patient is taken into care. If the patient has fallen, avoid lifting him/her unaided if injury is suspected, but secure him/her by ensuring a safe environment (removal of dangerous objects, protection against a further fall) is essential.

In the event of discomfort during home dialysis, it may be necessary to **check the medical equipment**. For example, in the event of suspected fluid imbalance or a problem with the catheter, you need to ensure that the treatment in progress (such as peritoneal dialysis) is correctly stopped or monitored, without handling the equipment inappropriately.

Prepare medical information and materials

While waiting for help to arrive, it's a good idea to have essential **medical information ready**, such as the patient's medication, medical history and latest test results (blood test, blood pressure, etc.). Having this information at hand enables the doctor or nurse to make rapid, informed decisions. This also includes preparing the patient's dialysis card or medical prescriptions.

If the patient is on dialysis, it's important to have clear information about the last session (date, duration, complications) and to note any abnormalities that appeared during the procedure.

- **Supporting the team in critical situations**: communication and stress management.

Communication and **stress management** are profoundly linked and essential, particularly in the healthcare field. Whether for caregivers, patients or relatives, effective communication helps to prevent misunderstandings, improve the quality of care, and ease the emotional tensions often present in the context of chronic illness or emergency situations. At the same time, stress management, both for healthcare professionals and for patients and their families, plays a key role in overall well-being and effective care. The way in which stress is managed, partly through communication, directly influences emotional state, decision-making and the quality of interpersonal relationships in these often difficult contexts.

The importance of clear, benevolent communication

Clear, benevolent communication is essential in medical care, as it creates a bond of trust between patient, caregiver and family. When patients understand what is happening to them, the treatments they are being offered, and the procedures to be followed, they are more likely to be involved in their own care, and to participate actively in the decisions that concern them. Fluid communication also reduces the risk of misunderstandings or medical errors, which is essential in a healthcare environment.

For caregivers, knowing how to **listen to** the patient is the first step to successful communication. Active listening, which involves paying attention to what the patient has to say without interrupting, and rephrasing to check for understanding, ensures that the patient feels heard. This is particularly crucial in stressful situations, where the person may find it difficult to express their concerns or needs clearly. For example, a dialysis patient may feel fear or anxiety about his or her treatment, and be reluctant to talk about it. Creating an environment of trust, where talking is encouraged and valued, makes it easier to tackle these sensitive subjects.

Clear explanations are also essential. For the patient, medical vocabulary can be a source of confusion and anxiety, especially when complex terms are used. It is important to adapt the language used so that it is understandable, without minimizing the seriousness of the situation. Giving simple explanations and checking that the patient has understood the information conveyed is essential to avoid misunderstandings that could generate stress or anxiety. This approach must also include the family or caregivers, who play a key role in supporting the patient.

The role of communication in stress management

The way in which communication is managed in a medical context plays a crucial role in stress management, for both patients and caregivers. For patients, receiving clear information tailored to their situation helps **reduce uncertainty**, which is one of the main sources of stress. Uncertainty linked to a chronic illness, a complex treatment or the evolution of one's health can provoke great anxiety. By explaining the next steps, clarifying treatment options, and offering a space to ask questions, patients can regain a form of control over their situation, which naturally alleviates stress.

Communication also plays a major role in managing emotions. When stress builds up, emotions can become difficult to manage, and patients may experience feelings of frustration, anger or despair. A caregiver who communicates with **empathy** can help defuse these negative emotions by acknowledging and validating them. Telling a patient "I understand how difficult this situation is for you" or "It's normal to be worried in this context" can ease much of their anxiety. It shows that their emotions are legitimate, and that they are not alone in going through this ordeal.

For caregivers themselves, **communication within the medical team** is essential to managing their own stress. Working in a healthcare environment, particularly in nephrology, can be very stressful due to heavy responsibilities, frequent medical emergencies, and the emotional burden of caring for patients with chronic illnesses. Good communication within the team helps to share this load, coordinate care effectively, and avoid situations where stress could lead to errors or misunderstandings. Discussing complex cases, helping each other out in the face of difficulties, and sharing informal moments of exchange help to strengthen cohesion and reduce the pressure felt.

Stress management techniques for caregivers and patients

Stress, whether felt by patients or caregivers, can be reduced through simple, accessible techniques. Learning to manage stress is an integral part of the care process, as poorly managed stress can adversely affect patient health and the quality of care provided.

For **patients**, stress can be linked to fear of the future, pain, or the uncertainty of treatment. Techniques such as **deep breathing**, **meditation** or **progressive relaxation** can help them to calm their minds and regain a sense of calm, particularly before or after a dialysis session, or in the recovery period after a transplant. These techniques help to relax the body and mind, by activating the parasympathetic nervous system, which counteracts the physiological effects of stress.

Positive visualization is another technique that can help patients manage anxiety. It involves imagining pleasant scenarios or projecting oneself into a situation where one feels safe and relaxed. This type of mental exercise diverts the patient's attention from immediate concerns and anchors them in a more serene state. Caregivers can also suggest that patients keep a **diary** to express their emotions and fears, which can have a cathartic and liberating effect.

For **caregivers**, stress management involves similar approaches, but adapted to their work context. **Colleague support** is crucial to creating a working environment where stress is recognized and dealt with collectively. Care teams can organize debriefing sessions after particularly stressful situations, to enable everyone to share their feelings and better digest the emotional burden. Mindfulness **meditation** is also increasingly recognized in medical circles as an effective method for reducing stress and increasing concentration and resilience in high-pressure situations.

In addition, caregivers need to learn to recognize the **warning signs of burn-out**, such as chronic fatigue, irritability, or loss of interest in work. When these signs appear, it's essential to **step back**, delegate some responsibilities if possible, and seek support. Caregivers' well-being is essential to the quality of care they provide, and that means managing their own stress and emotions.

Creating a soothing communication environment

Finally, the way in which the work or care environment is structured influences communication and stress management. In a hospital or dialysis center, it's important to create a **reassuring environment** for patients, where they feel listened to and supported. A calm environment, with respectful, caring exchanges between caregivers and patients, naturally reduces stress levels. Using simple words, asking open-ended questions, and offering pauses in discussions helps maintain calm communication.

Non-verbal communication gestures also play an important role. A smile, benevolent eye contact or an open posture can ease tension and reinforce a sense of trust and security. It's important to remember that communication is not just about words, but also about the caregiver's overall attitude towards the patient.

Chapter 11

Pain management in nephrology

- **Types of pain specific to kidney disease**: Pain associated with renal colic, arteriovenous fistulas, etc.

The pain associated with renal colic and arteriovenous fistulas is particularly intense, and requires appropriate management to relieve the patient while preventing possible complications. Although different in nature and origin, these pains share an acute, often unpredictable character, and can severely impair the patient's quality of life. Understanding these pains, their mechanisms, and management strategies is essential to offer rapid and effective relief, while avoiding sequelae or inappropriate treatment.

The pain of renal colic: an emergency that must be managed quickly

Renal colic is one of the most intense forms of pain you can experience. It is caused by a kidney stone that obstructs the urinary tract, usually the ureter, preventing the normal flow of urine. This obstruction creates pressure upstream, leading to dilatation of the renal cavities and inflammation that irritates the nerve endings. The pain, often described as "unbearable", is generally **acute, localized in the flank**, and may radiate to the abdomen, groin or genitals.

The main characteristic of renal colic pain is its **paroxysmal nature**. It comes on suddenly, often without warning, with intense peaks followed by phases of respite of varying duration. This phenomenon is explained by the contractions of the urinary tract as it attempts to dislodge the stone. Patients may also experience nausea, vomiting and restlessness, in contrast to other abdominal pains which often lead to immobility.

Pain management for renal colic is based on the use of **powerful analgesics**, notably non-steroidal anti-inflammatory drugs (NSAIDs), which reduce inflammation and swelling in the urinary tract, thus facilitating the flow of urine. **Antispasmodics** are also used to reduce contractions of the smooth muscles of the ureter. In the most severe cases, where pain does not respond to these treatments, opioids may be administered. Rapid pain relief is crucial to prevent dehydration and fatigue due to the intensity of the attack.

In addition to immediate pain management, long-term management is needed to prevent the formation of new stones and recurrence of renal colic. This includes **regular monitoring**, dietary advice (particularly on hydration and reducing the intake of certain oxalate-rich foods), and specific treatments to dissolve or eliminate existing stones.

Pain associated with arteriovenous fistulas: chronic discomfort to monitor

The **arteriovenous fistula (AVF)** is a vascular access created surgically to enable dialysis in patients with kidney failure. It connects an artery to a vein, thereby increasing the blood flow required for filtration. Although the fistula is essential for dialysis treatment, it can cause chronic or acute pain in some patients.

Pain associated with an arteriovenous fistula can have several causes. In the days or weeks following the creation of the fistula, it is normal to feel **discomfort linked to healing**, inflammation and the adaptation of the blood vessels to this new connection. This pain is often moderate and transient, and can be relieved by **mild analgesics** such as paracetamol. However, if the pain persists or intensifies, it may indicate complications such as **thrombosis**, **infection** or **stenosis** (narrowing of the vessel), requiring immediate medical attention.

Chronic discomfort can also be caused by repeated **fistula puncture** sessions. Each dialysis session requires two punctures of the fistula to enable connection to the extracorporeal circuit, which can lead to increased sensitivity and local pain, especially if the skin becomes fragile. In such cases, it is essential to educate patients on how to maintain their fistula to minimize the risk of infection and pain. The application of **anesthetic creams** prior to puncture can help reduce perceived pain, while the use of **strict hygiene techniques** can reduce the risk of complications.

If a fistula becomes continuously painful, with **abnormal noise** (change in fistula murmur), **swelling** or **local heat**, this may be a sign of a serious vascular complication, such as thrombosis or aneurysm. In such cases, prompt intervention is crucial to preserve fistula functionality and avoid potentially serious infection.

Post-operative pain after kidney transplantation: recovery after major surgery

Kidney transplantation is a major surgical procedure that enables patients suffering from end-stage renal failure to regain normal kidney function. However, post-operative recovery can be accompanied by pain, particularly in the abdomen, where the transplanted kidney is implanted. Post-operative pain is generally due to tissue healing and surgical manipulation, and can last for several weeks after the operation.

These pains are usually **well controlled** with standard analgesics, and their intensity diminishes over time. However, persistent pain or worsening discomfort may be a sign of complications, such as **inflammation of the graft**, **infection**, or problems related to healing (such as a hernia). Regular monitoring for signs of infection (fever, redness, heat around the scar) is therefore essential.

Patients should be informed that **moderate pain** is normal for the first few weeks after transplantation, but should gradually subside. Pain medication should be adapted to the intensity of the pain, taking care to avoid non-steroidal anti-inflammatory drugs, which may be contraindicated in transplant patients due to their effects on renal function.

Pain associated with dialysis treatment: a daily discomfort to manage

Dialysis treatments, whether hemodialysis or peritoneal dialysis, can sometimes cause pain. In hemodialysis, pain is often associated with the creation and puncture of the fistula, as mentioned above, but it can also result from muscle cramps, which are common in dialysis patients due to the rapid changes in fluid and electrolyte levels during sessions.

These **muscle cramps** can be very painful and are often felt in the legs. They are generally due to sodium or potassium imbalances, or to too rapid a reduction in blood volume during dialysis. Adjustments to the dialysis treatment, such as a more gradual reduction of excess fluid, may be necessary to reduce their frequency and intensity. **Gentle stretching** and the application of local heat can also help relieve these pains after the session.

In the case of **peritoneal dialysis**, pain may be related to the introduction of dialysis fluid into the abdomen, which may cause a sensation of abdominal pressure or distension. Pain is often transient, but if it persists or worsens, it may indicate a peritoneal infection (peritonitis), requiring urgent medical attention.

- **Pain assessment scales**: Techniques for assessing pain in patients.

Assessing a patient's pain is a crucial step in medical management, particularly in patients with chronic kidney disease or those on dialysis, who may experience various forms of pain, whether acute or chronic. Proper pain assessment is essential to adapt treatment, provide effective relief and prevent complications. However, since pain is a subjective experience, it can be difficult to quantify. Caregivers must therefore use rigorous assessment techniques, including observation, dialogue and standardized tools, to better understand the intensity, location and nature of the pain experienced by the patient.

The importance of a global, empathetic approach

Before discussing specific pain assessment techniques, it is essential to understand that the approach must be **global and empathic**. Pain is a multifactorial experience, influenced by physical, emotional and psychological factors. A patient suffering from kidney disease may experience pain not only because of his or her pathology, but also because of anxiety, fears or the frustration associated with chronic illness.

Caregivers must therefore adopt an **active, sympathetic** listening **posture** when questioning patients about their pain. Creating a climate of trust, where patients feel free to express themselves without judgment, is essential to obtaining accurate information. Many patients may minimize or, conversely, exaggerate their pain depending on their emotional state. By listening attentively and adopting an empathetic attitude, we can gather more reliable information and adapt our treatment accordingly.

Using pain scales: a standardized, objective tool

One of the most commonly used tools for assessing pain is the **pain assessment scale**, which quantifies the intensity of pain felt by the patient. Different scales are available, adapted to each patient's ability to understand and his or her needs, enabling a more precise assessment.

The simplest scale is the **numeric scale** (or EN), where the patient is asked to rate his or her pain on a scale from 0 to 10, with 0 representing the total absence of pain and 10 the most intense pain imaginable. This method is particularly useful for patients who are able to assess and verbalize their pain accurately. However, it is important to clearly explain how to use this scale, as some patients, particularly the elderly or those with cognitive impairments, may have difficulty interpreting it.

For patients who have difficulty using the numerical scale, other methods exist, such as the **Visual Analog Scale** (VAS), where the patient indicates their pain level on a horizontal line, or the **Simple Verbal Scale** (SVS), where they are asked to qualify their pain with terms such as "none", "mild", "moderate" or "intense". These methods offer more concrete benchmarks for patients who have difficulty expressing the intensity of their pain numerically.

Face scales (such as the Wong-Baker scale) are useful for children, the elderly or those with cognitive difficulties. This scale presents faces ranging from a smiling face to a very sad or crying face, and the patient selects the face that best reflects his or her feelings. It's an effective technique for people who have difficulty verbalizing their pain.

Qualitative pain assessment: understanding the nature and characteristics of pain

In addition to the intensity of the pain, it's important to assess its **qualitative characteristics**. Pain can be sharp, dull, stabbing, acute or chronic, and these descriptions can give valuable clues as to the origin of the pain. Asking the patient about the **nature of** the pain helps us to better understand the underlying mechanisms and adapt treatment.

For example, **sudden stabbing** pain, often felt in the flank or radiating to the groin, typically suggests renal colic caused by a kidney stone, while **chronic, dull** pain around the site of an arteriovenous fistula may indicate a vascular problem or edema. **Sharp, burning** pain in the abdomen after peritoneal dialysis may suggest peritonitis.

It's also important to ask the patient what factors **trigger** or **relieve** pain. Some pains may be exacerbated by movement or a particular position (as in the case of a painful fistula), while others, such as muscle cramps during dialysis, may be relieved by a change of position or light massage. Asking questions about the evolution of pain over time, its rhythms (for example, more intense pain at night), and its impact on the patient's day-to-day life, helps to build a more complete picture.

Observation: a valuable tool for assessing pain in non-verbal patients

In certain situations, patients may be unable to verbalize their pain, due to an altered state of consciousness, cognitive difficulties or neurological disorders. In such cases, **observing physical signs** becomes an indispensable tool for assessing pain. Caregivers need to be alert to a number of non-verbal cues that may signal significant pain, including **facial expressions** (grimacing, tensing up), **body movements** (agitation, protection of a body part, sudden withdrawal), or **changes in behavior** (aggression, withdrawal, confusion).

Physiological signs can also indicate intense pain: increased heart rate (tachycardia), raised blood pressure, rapid, shallow breathing (polypnoea), or excessive sweating. These signs should be taken into account, especially in frail patients or those unable to express themselves, as they may signal a level of pain that requires urgent intervention.

In contexts where the patient is unconscious or unable to communicate, specific scales, such as the **Behavioral Pain Scale (BPS)**, can be used. These scales assess pain according to the patient's behavioral responses to stimuli or manipulations, such as touch, change of position or care. These tools enable pain to be measured objectively and analgesic treatments to be adjusted more precisely.

Regular pain re-evaluation: an essential follow-up

Pain assessment is not limited to a single measurement, but must be carried out **regularly and repeatedly**. Pain can change over time, depending on the patient's treatment or state of health. Once a treatment has been put in place, it is essential to **reassess pain** at

144

regular intervals to ensure that the measures taken are effective and that the patient is relieved. If the pain persists or worsens, it may be necessary to readjust the treatment, propose an alternative therapy or consider further tests to investigate the underlying cause.

In addition, regular assessment enables us to verify the impact of treatment on the patient's quality of life. Well-managed pain allows patients to regain greater autonomy, sleep better and maintain a stable emotional state. Questions about a **return to normal activity** or **changes in sleep patterns may** indicate an overall improvement in the patient's well-being, over and above simple pain relief.

Take into account the emotional and psychological context of pain

Pain, especially chronic pain, can have a **major psychological impact** on the patient. Anxiety, depression or stress can amplify the perception of pain, making it more difficult to tolerate. It is therefore important to take these emotional factors into account when assessing pain, and to discuss these aspects with the patient.

Asking the patient about his or her **emotional state**, fears or worries related to pain may reveal aggravating factors. In some cases, a multidisciplinary approach, including psychological support, may be required to help the patient manage pain more effectively and regain mental equilibrium. Pain should never be seen in isolation, but rather as a global experience, influenced by physical, emotional and social factors.

- **Non-medication management**: Emotional support, relaxation techniques, comfortable positions.

Emotional support, **relaxation techniques** and the choice of **comfortable positions** are essential elements in improving the quality of life of patients with chronic illnesses, and in particular those suffering from kidney disease. These complementary approaches aim not only to relieve physical symptoms, but also to reduce the stress, anxiety and psychological suffering that can accompany the disease. Emotional support enables patients to feel listened to and understood, while relaxation techniques and comfortable positions help to soothe the body and mind, promoting better tolerance of treatment and overall well-being.

Emotional support: attentive, empathetic listening

Emotional support is an essential component of care for patients with kidney disease, especially those on dialysis or after transplantation. Faced with the chronicity of the disease, uncertainties about the future, and the burdensome nature of treatment, patients can experience feelings of discouragement, anxiety and even depression. The role of caregivers and loved ones is to provide a space where patients can **express their fears, doubts and frustrations**, without fear of being judged or misunderstood.

The first element of emotional support is **active listening**. This means being fully present when the patient speaks, without interrupting, while showing that his or her feelings are understood and taken into account. Active listening can take the form of verbal cues, such as rephrasing what the patient has said to check for understanding, but also non-verbal cues, such as sympathetic eye contact or a nod of the head. It's essential not to minimize the patient's concerns, even if they seem irrational or exaggerated. A phrase like "I understand that this situation is difficult for you" or "It's normal to feel worried in these circumstances" can already bring great relief, by validating the patient's emotions.

Beyond listening, emotional support can also include **practical advice** to help patients better manage the psychological aspects of their illness. For example, encouraging patients to talk about their concerns with someone close to them, or referring them to a **psychologist** or support group, can help them feel less isolated. These spaces enable patients to share their experiences with others in similar situations, which can be extremely reassuring and calming.

Relaxation techniques: calming body and mind

Relaxation techniques are a valuable tool for helping patients manage the stress and anxiety that often accompany a chronic illness such as kidney failure. Relaxation helps to reduce physical tension, calm the nervous system and soothe the mind, creating a virtuous circle where body and mind support each other.

Deep breathing is one of the simplest and most accessible relaxation techniques. It re-establishes a soothing breathing rhythm and oxygenates the body in depth. When patients feel anxious or in pain, they can be guided to practice slow, deep breathing. Inhaling deeply through the nose to the count of 4, then exhaling slowly through the mouth to the count of 4 again, helps activate the parasympathetic nervous system, which is responsible for relaxation. This exercise can be performed at any time, and its immediate effect on reducing anxiety is often noticeable.

Guided meditation is another effective relaxation technique, particularly for patients who find it difficult to relax. It involves focusing attention on soothing thoughts or positive mental images, often under the guidance of a caregiver or via a meditation app. By focusing on a reassuring voice that guides their breathing and attention, patients can gradually push away negative or anxious thoughts and immerse themselves in a deeper state of relaxation.

Progressive muscle relaxation exercises are also very useful for relieving body tension, which can build up as a result of chronic pain or stress. This technique involves successively contracting and releasing different muscle groups, starting with the feet and gradually working up to the head. By concentrating on each part of the body, patients become more aware of their muscular tensions and learn to release them, which can lead to a reduction in physical pain and better overall relaxation.

Comfortable positions: relieve pain and promote rest

Choosing **comfortable positions** is particularly important for patients with kidney disease, as many suffer chronic pain or discomfort related to complications such as renal colic, arteriovenous fistula or dialysis sequelae. Finding the right position not only relieves pain, but also facilitates breathing and promotes restful sleep, which is essential for the patient's well-being.

In the case of renal colic pain, for example, a semi-seated or **lateral decubitus** position (lying on one side) can help reduce pressure on the kidneys and relieve spasms. It is also useful to offer the patient **support cushions** to maintain a comfortable posture and avoid muscular tension. Caregivers can adjust the patient's position regularly to prevent pain associated with prolonged immobility and avoid pressure points that could lead to pressure sores.

For patients with **arteriovenous fistulas**, it is crucial to avoid compressing the arm where the fistula is placed. Positions that allow the arm to be held in a slightly elevated posture, supported by a pillow, can reduce the discomfort associated with repeated punctures or vascular complications. Particular attention should be paid to immobilizing the arm during dialysis sessions, and the patient should be encouraged to gently move his or her fingers to promote circulation without affecting the fistula.

Finally, lying down or semi-seated positions are also beneficial for patients suffering from **respiratory difficulties** linked to pulmonary edema or fluid overload. The semi-seated position facilitates breathing by reducing pressure on the diaphragm and lungs, while improving oxygenation. This position is particularly recommended during attacks of dyspnea, or during episodes of fluid overload after a dialysis session.

Chapter 12

Technological innovation in nephrology

- **New technologies for monitoring and treating kidney patients**: home dialysis, telemedicine, applications for monitoring vital signs.

Home dialysis, telemedicine and patient monitoring applications represent major technological and organizational advances in the care of patients suffering from chronic renal failure. These innovations enable greater patient autonomy, personalized care and improved quality of life. They also mark a shift towards connected medicine, where patients are more involved in their treatment, while benefiting from rigorous remote medical monitoring. These approaches offer alternatives to traditional hospital care, while ensuring the safety and efficacy of treatments.

Home dialysis: autonomy and improved quality of life

Home dialysis, whether hemodialysis or peritoneal dialysis, has become an increasingly popular solution for patients suffering from chronic renal failure. It offers an alternative to regular dialysis center sessions, enabling patients to carry out their treatment in the comfort of their own home. This offers many advantages, including greater flexibility in treatment management, reduced travel and time spent in healthcare facilities, and improved quality of life.

In **home hemodialysis**, a hemodialysis machine is installed in the patient's home. The patient, often assisted by a trained family member, learns to perform the sessions himself, prepare the equipment, insert the needles into the arteriovenous fistula, and monitor the parameters during the session. This option allows patients to choose their own schedule and adapt the frequency of sessions to their needs, often with more frequent but shorter sessions. This makes dialysis gentler and better tolerated by the body. Home hemodialysis also offers psychological comfort, as the patient is in a familiar environment, surrounded by loved ones.

Home peritoneal dialysis is another popular option. This method uses the peritoneum, the membrane surrounding the abdominal organs, as a filter to remove toxins and excess fluid from the body. The patient fills the abdominal cavity with a dialysis solution via an implanted catheter, allows the solution to act for several hours, then empties it. This process can be carried out manually several times a day (continuous ambulatory peritoneal dialysis) or automatically overnight using a machine (automated peritoneal dialysis). This type of dialysis offers great freedom to the patient, who can continue his or her daily activities without being interrupted by dialysis sessions in a center.

Patient training is a key element in the success of home dialysis. Caregivers train patients and their families to use the equipment safely, to recognize the signs of complications (such as infections or problems with the fistula or catheter), and to react in the event of a problem. Regular follow-up is provided, and in case of doubt, patients can contact their medical team. This enhanced autonomy contributes to **improved quality of life**, as patients become active players in their treatment, with greater flexibility and more direct control over their care.

Telemedicine: enhanced remote medical monitoring

Telemedicine has become an essential tool in the management of chronic diseases such as kidney failure. It enables patients undergoing dialysis at home, or those with regular follow-up needs, to benefit from medical supervision without having to travel to the hospital or dialysis center. This is particularly beneficial for patients living in rural or remote areas, where access to nephrology specialists may be limited.

Thanks to telemedicine, patients can have **remote consultations** with their nephrologist or healthcare team. These consultations, carried out by videoconference or telephone, enable them to discuss test results, adjust treatment, or ask questions about symptoms or doubts concerning dialysis. Telemedicine also offers the possibility of **sharing data in real time**, thanks in particular to applications for monitoring vitals or the connected devices used during dialysis sessions. This enables the doctor to proactively monitor the patient's state of health and intervene quickly if necessary.

Telemedicine also helps **reduce stress** for patients, as they can get quick answers to their questions without waiting for a physical consultation. It also helps maintain a relationship of trust with the healthcare team, even at a distance. Telemedicine consultations can be scheduled on a regular basis to monitor disease progression and adjust treatments, but they are also useful in emergencies, to avoid unnecessary travel or hospitalization.

One of the main advantages of telemedicine is the possibility of **multidisciplinary follow-up** at a distance. Patients can talk to their nephrologist, but also to dieticians, psychologists or specialized nurses, depending on their needs. This coordination of care ensures comprehensive management, with every aspect of the patient's health monitored consistently and proactively.

Applications for monitoring vital signs: the era of connected health

Constant monitoring applications and connected devices are an integral part of telemedicine and chronic disease management in the home. These tools enable patients to monitor key health parameters in real time, such as blood pressure, weight, heart rate, and blood glucose or potassium levels. This data is then automatically transmitted to the care team, who can monitor the patient's health and intervene if any anomalies are detected.

In home dialysis, **vitals monitoring applications** play a crucial role in monitoring indicators such as **fluid balance**, an essential parameter for preventing fluid overload or dehydration. By recording their weight on a daily basis and monitoring the volumes of fluid eliminated during dialysis sessions, patients can, with the help of their doctor, adjust their treatment according to their needs.

These applications can also integrate **treatment reminders**, to ensure that patients take their medication on time and comply with dialysis protocols. Patients can also receive notifications prompting them to follow specific dietary advice or exercise. This helps them stay more engaged and better understand the impact of their lifestyle on their health.

One of the great advantages of connected health applications is that they facilitate **real-time communication with** the healthcare team. If an abnormal variation is detected (for example, sudden hypertension or rapid weight gain suggesting fluid retention), the system can alert the doctor or nurse, who can contact the patient to assess the situation and take action. This enables more reactive and preventive management, avoiding serious complications or emergency hospitalization.

What's more, monitoring applications enable patients to **visualize the evolution of their health** through graphs or dashboards, which can be highly motivating. Patients become more aware of the links between their daily habits (diet, physical activity, hydration) and their state of health, which helps them to better manage their disease in the long term.

- **The impact of robotization and artificial intelligence**: decision-making tools, impact on the nursing profession.

Decision-support tools have become key elements in care practice, providing invaluable support to healthcare professionals, including caregivers, in their day-to-day work. These tools, often integrated into IT systems, mobile applications or telemedicine devices, help to improve the quality of care, facilitate complex decision-making and optimize patient management. They influence not only the work of nurses and doctors, but also that of care assistants, modifying their practices and offering them new opportunities to participate in more comprehensive, personalized care.

Decision support tools: technological support for care

Decision support tools are digital systems designed to assist caregivers in patient management, by providing recommendations or alerts based on collected health data. They are based on **algorithms** and medical databases that analyze patient-related information (such as vital signs, test results and medical history) in real time. These tools are used to **facilitate decision-making** in complex clinical situations, by proposing adapted solutions or treatment paths to follow, according to the patient's needs.

These tools are also capable of **detecting early anomalies** in a patient's state of health, well before clinical symptoms appear. For example, a system can alert the care team to the detection of abnormally low blood pressure or high potassium levels, factors that may indicate a risk of decompensation or a potential complication in patients with renal failure. Healthcare professionals can then intervene rapidly to adjust treatment or propose specific care.

For caregivers, these tools enable **better anticipation of** patient needs. They provide valuable information on the evolution of health parameters, facilitating daily care. For example, thanks to decision-support tools, a caregiver can receive alerts indicating that a patient's diuresis is insufficient, signalling possible fluid retention that requires further assessment. This early detection helps prevent serious complications such as pulmonary oedema or hypervolaemia, which are common risks in dialysis patients.

In addition to providing information on a patient's current state of health, decision-support tools also enable **data** to **be centralized** and easily accessed. The caregiver can, for example, consult the latest results of biological tests, medical prescriptions, or a patient's history via a digital interface, enabling care to be adapted more effectively and ensuring better continuity of care, in collaboration with other team members.

Impact on the nursing profession: greater autonomy and a more proactive approach

The integration of decision-support tools into the practice of nursing assistants has a significant impact on their role and responsibilities. Although they remain within a care framework focused on assisting patients and supporting nurses, these tools enable them to **gain autonomy** and play a more active role in overall patient care.

Traditionally, the caregiver's role has been to provide basic care (such as grooming, mobilization, feeding assistance) and monitor basic clinical signs, such as temperature or diuresis. With the advent of decision-support tools, their role has expanded, as they can now **monitor more detailed data**, such as vital parameters or test results, placing them at the heart of more advanced and responsive monitoring. For example, a caregiver working with dialysis patients can receive notifications of anomalies in dialysis results, and quickly inform the medical team or adjust care accordingly.

These tools also make it possible to **delegate certain** routine **care decisions** to caregivers, while remaining within a reassuring framework. For example, if a patient experiences a drop in blood pressure in connection with a treatment or dialysis session, a decision support tool can suggest a series of actions to be taken (such as placing the patient in a recumbent position with legs elevated, or administering a fluid intake), which the caregiver can carry out in complete safety. This type of decision-making, based on real-time data, strengthens their ability **to react appropriately and autonomously**.

Another notable impact of decision-support tools is to **reduce the risk of errors** in routine care. For example, caregivers, when managing medication or taking part in simple medical procedures, can be guided by real-time alerts that warn them of incorrect doses or medical contraindications. This improves patient safety and enables the caregiver to work with greater confidence and precision.

Improving interprofessional collaboration

Decision-support tools also promote **better inter-professional collaboration**. By centralizing data and giving every member of the care team access to the same information, they facilitate communication between the various professionals involved in a patient's care. As a result, caregivers can better coordinate their actions with those of nurses, doctors and other healthcare professionals, ensuring a more harmonious and efficient approach to care.

For example, a caregiver can quickly pass on important information to nurses or doctors based on data collected via a decision-support tool. If a patient shows signs of dehydration or edema after a dialysis session, the caregiver can immediately report the anomaly to the medical team, who can take the necessary measures, such as adjusting the volume of fluid extracted during subsequent sessions. This fluidity in the transmission of information helps avoid delays in treatment and improves clinical outcomes.

What's more, caregivers can also better understand **medical decisions** thanks to these tools. By accessing medical records and treatment recommendations in real time, they can adapt their care in a way that is more relevant and aligned with the medical team's objectives. This reinforces their role within the care team, and allows them to be more involved in collective decision-making processes, particularly during care coordination meetings.

Training and adaptation to the new technological environment

With the introduction of decision-support tools into their practice, caregivers also need **appropriate training** to familiarize them with these technologies. Although these tools are designed to be simple to use, initial training is essential to enable caregivers to fully understand how they work and make the most of them.

This training must include not only technical aspects, such as how to enter and interpret data, but also **communication** and emergency management **skills**. Indeed, caregivers need to know how to react in the event of an alert or anomaly detected by the tool, and be able to communicate this information effectively to other members of the care team.

The introduction of decision-support tools is also changing the way caregivers deal with **technology** in their day-to-day work. They must learn to integrate these tools into their routine without losing human contact with the patient, as the relational aspect remains a fundamental element of their profession. The use of technology should not replace the need to listen and listen to the patient, but rather enable them to better anticipate his or her needs and offer more personalized, tailored care.

- **Training in new technologies**: The caregiver and technological developments in the sector.

As a key player in the care process, the nursing auxiliary is today confronted with **technological developments** that are profoundly transforming the healthcare sector. These advances affect working methods, the tools used and the organization of care. While these technologies bring many advantages, they are also revolutionizing the practice of nursing assistants, who must adapt to these changes while maintaining their fundamental role of being close to patients and providing them with support. The integration of new technologies, such as telemedicine, connected devices, electronic medical records and decision-support tools, is changing caregivers' day-to-day tasks, while offering opportunities to improve the quality of care.

A changing role: greater autonomy and responsibility

With the advent of new technologies, the role of the nursing auxiliary is expanding and becoming more complex. Care assistants are no longer solely responsible for **basic care**, such as hygiene, feeding and mobilizing patients. Thanks to digital devices and decision-support tools, they are now more actively involved in **clinical monitoring of** patients, collecting and analyzing health data, and communicating with the medical team.

For example, the use of **connected devices** enables caregivers to monitor patients' vital signs in real time. This means they can be at the forefront of detecting anomalies, such as variations in blood pressure, oxygen saturation or weight, which may indicate a potential complication. These devices give caregivers greater **autonomy in decision-making**, as they can react quickly by adjusting care or alerting the nursing or medical team before a situation worsens.

In addition, caregivers are increasingly involved in the use of **digital care monitoring tools**, such as electronic medical records (EMRs), which centralize all information concerning a patient. Thanks to these tools, they can easily access care histories, prescriptions and health check-ups, enabling them to tailor their interventions to the patient's current needs. This centralization of data makes communication with other healthcare professionals smoother, and ensures **continuity of care** with no break in information.

Training and adapting to new technologies: an unavoidable challenge

The integration of new technologies into the day-to-day work of nurses' aides means a greater need for **training** and adaptation. To be fully effective, these digital tools require caregivers to master the basics of how they work. While some technologies, such as tablets or vital signs monitors, are relatively intuitive, other tools, such as care management software or remote monitoring applications, require more in-depth training.

Caregivers therefore need to develop new skills, particularly in **IT and data management**, to understand and use these devices correctly. It is essential to provide them with appropriate **educational support**, with ongoing training to keep them up to date with rapidly evolving technologies. This is not just limited to the technical use of tools, but also includes notions of **data security** and **confidentiality**, as caregivers handle sensitive medical information in digital systems.

In addition, training must also include more technical aspects related to the **specific pathologies** that caregivers may encounter. For example, in the case of renal failure, caregivers can be trained in the use of remote monitoring devices that track parameters related to dialysis or to potential complications of this pathology, such as hyperkalemia or pulmonary edema. By acquiring this expertise, care assistants become key players in monitoring the health of patients at home or in care centers.

A patient-caregiver relationship strengthened by technology

Although technologies are introducing digital tools into everyday care, the human role of the caregiver, as the **pillar of the patient-caregiver relationship**, remains central. Indeed, caregivers are often the professionals closest to patients, those with whom they interact most frequently. They are at the heart of **emotional support**, listening, and accompaniment in daily care. These relational aspects do not disappear with the arrival of technology; on the contrary, they are reinforced.

Digital devices and connected tools **free up** caregivers' **time** to focus more on relational care. For example, by automating certain administrative tasks or simplifying clinical data collection, caregivers can focus on what's essential: accompanying the patient, listening to his or her needs, and observing his or her emotional state. These technologies also offer greater flexibility in work organization, enabling better management of the time spent with each patient.

In telemedicine, where remote consultations are becoming increasingly common, nursing assistants can act as **mediators between** patient and doctor. They can accompany patients during online consultations, helping them to prepare, ensuring that all parameters are properly monitored, and above all, explaining medical recommendations to patients and assisting them in implementing prescribed treatments. This close relationship is all the more valuable as some patients, particularly the elderly, may be disoriented or anxious about using technology. The caregiver then becomes a reassuring figure, able to **bridge the gap between technological innovations and human needs**.

The challenge of humanization in a technological environment

Although technology brings considerable benefits in terms of care efficiency and safety, a major challenge for caregivers is to **maintain a human approach in an increasingly digital environment**. There is a risk that excessive use of technology can, in some cases, create a distance between caregiver and patient, especially if attention is diverted to screens and connected devices.

It is therefore essential that caregivers learn to **integrate technology harmoniously** into their practice, while not losing sight of the importance of human contact. Digital devices must be seen as tools for care, not as replacements for human interaction. For example, when taking vital signs or performing clinical monitoring using connected devices, the caregiver can take advantage of these moments to engage in conversation with the patient, reassure him or her, and observe his or her general state beyond simple medical parameters.

Care must always include an **emotional and relational dimension**, even in a technological context. The look, the touch, the words of encouragement and attentive listening are aspects that technology cannot replace. In this sense, caregivers have a fundamental role to play in **humanizing technology** and ensuring that innovations do not create a barrier between the patient and healthcare professionals, but on the contrary, enhance their interaction and mutual understanding.

Towards a future of connected, personalized care

Technological developments in the healthcare sector offer **promising prospects** for improving the quality and personalization of care. The future of connected care, with telemedicine devices, biometric sensors and remote monitoring applications, paves the way for more **individualized** patient management, with care adjusted in real time to each patient's specific needs. For caregivers, this means they will have access to a multitude of tools enabling them to better understand the evolution of their patients' state of health, and to respond rapidly to warning signals.

The development of **predictive healthcare**, where data analysis can anticipate complications even before symptoms appear, will strengthen the role of caregivers in the prevention and early detection of health problems. Thanks to ongoing training and the integration of technology into their practice, they will be able to play a more active part in this evolution towards proactive, personalized medicine.

Chapter 13

Pediatric nephrology: specific care for children

- **Common pediatric renal pathologies**: Nephrotic syndrome, acute renal failure in children.

Nephrotic syndrome and **acute renal failure)ARF)** in children are two serious renal conditions that require rapid and appropriate management. Although they may have different origins, they share common features, including a major impact on renal function and significant consequences for the child's fluid and electrolyte balance. Understanding these two conditions, their manifestations, treatments and specific implications in children is essential to improve prognosis and prevent complications.

Nephrotic syndrome in children: protein loss and fluid imbalance

Nephrotic syndrome in children is a renal pathology characterized by excessive protein leakage into the urine (proteinuria), resulting from impaired filtration function of the renal glomeruli. This loss of proteins, particularly albumin, leads to a series of imbalances that affect the whole body. The causes of nephrotic syndrome can be varied, but in children, the most frequent form is **idiopathic nephrotic syndrome**, i.e. without a precise identified cause, often linked to minimal abnormalities of the glomeruli (minimal injury disease).

Massive proteinuria is the key sign of nephrotic syndrome, with large quantities of protein eliminated in the urine. This leads to **hypoalbuminemia**, a decrease in albumin levels in the blood, responsible for a reduction in oncotic pressure. As a result, fluid leaves the blood vessels and accumulates in the tissues, causing **edema** often visible in the face, legs, feet and abdomen (ascites). These edemas can be very marked and develop rapidly, sometimes overnight, causing significant discomfort for the child, with a puffy face in the morning or difficulty in walking due to swelling of the feet and legs.

In addition to edema, nephrotic syndrome exposes the child to increased risk of **complications**, such as infections, due to loss of immunoglobulins in the urine, and **thrombosis**, due to hypercoagulability caused by leakage of anticoagulant proteins. **Dyslipidemia** is also common, with increased levels of lipids in the blood, which is a compensatory response to protein loss.

Treatment of nephrotic syndrome in children relies mainly on **corticosteroids**, which are effective in the majority of cases. Steroid treatment aims to reduce inflammation of the glomeruli and halt protein loss in the urine. In around 80% of cases, children respond well to this treatment, with remission of proteinuria. However, some children may suffer **frequent relapses** or become **cortico-dependent** or **cortico-resistant**, requiring alternative immunosuppressive treatments.

Long-term follow-up is crucial, as nephrotic syndrome can evolve unpredictably. Parents need to be aware of warning signs, such as the return of edema, and know how to regularly monitor their child's urine to detect an early relapse. A low-salt diet is generally recommended to limit oedema, and strict monitoring of fluid and electrolyte balance is essential, as these children can easily become hypo- or hypervolaemic.

Acute renal failure in children: a medical emergency

Acute renal failure (ARF) in children is a condition in which the kidneys suddenly cease to function properly, resulting in an inability to filter waste products from the blood, regulate electrolytes and maintain fluid balance. Unlike chronic renal failure, which develops over a long period of time, AKI is a **medical emergency** that can occur rapidly and lead to serious, even fatal, complications if not treated immediately.

The causes of acute renal failure in children are manifold and can be classified into three categories: **pre-renal, renal and postrenal**.

- **Prerenal causes** are the most frequent and are linked to a decrease in renal perfusion, often caused by severe

165

dehydration, hypovolemic shock, or significant blood loss. In children, acute gastroenteritis with vomiting and severe diarrhea is a frequent cause of severe dehydration leading to acute renal failure.

- **Renal** (intrinsic) **causes** include direct damage to kidney tissue, for example as a result of acute glomerulonephritis, acute tubular necrosis or toxins. Severe infections or certain autoimmune diseases can also cause direct kidney damage.

- **Post-renal causes** result from an obstruction of the urinary tract, preventing the evacuation of urine. In infants and young children, congenital malformation of the urinary tract can lead to this type of renal failure.

The symptoms of ARF are generally those of **anuria** (absence of urine) or **oliguria** (severe reduction in urine production), associated with fluid retention in the body, which can lead to pulmonary edema, hypertension or cardiac disorders. Electrolyte disorders, particularly **hyperkalemia** (high potassium levels), are a major danger, as they can cause **heart rhythm disorders** leading to cardiac arrest. Other signs include drowsiness, apathy, fatigue, nausea and vomiting.

Diagnosis of acute renal failure is based on blood and urine tests, which reveal elevated **creatinine** and **urea** levels, as well as electrolyte imbalances. An ultrasound scan of the kidneys is often performed to look for obstruction or structural abnormalities.

Treatment of AKI depends on the underlying cause, but is generally aimed at **restoring renal perfusion**, correcting electrolyte imbalances, and treating acute complications. In children with acute pre-renal renal failure due to dehydration, **rapid rehydration** with intravenous solutions is often effective in restoring renal function. If severe hyperkalemia is present, urgent measures are needed to lower potassium levels, such as administration of **calcium gluconate**, **sodium bicarbonate**, or **ion-exchange resins**.

In cases of severe renal failure, or when initial treatments fail, **dialysis** may be required to temporarily replace kidney function until the kidneys recover. **Peritoneal dialysis** is often preferred in young children, as it is less invasive and easier to implement than hemodialysis. Management of AKI requires intensive monitoring to prevent complications, particularly pulmonary edema, infections and metabolic imbalances.

- **The role of the caregiver in the pediatric ward**: Specific support for children and their families.

Supporting children with kidney disease and their families is a complex and delicate process that goes far beyond medical care. It involves comprehensive physical, emotional and psychological care, because these illnesses - whether chronic disorders such as nephrotic syndrome, or acute pathologies such as acute renal failure - affect not only the child, but the whole family. The experience of illness, the management of heavy treatments such as dialysis or corticosteroid therapy, and uncertainty about the evolution of the child's health can be sources of stress, anxiety and fatigue for parents and siblings. The aim of specific support is therefore to offer adapted support at every stage of the illness, taking into account the individual needs of the child and his or her family environment.

Psychological and emotional guidance for children: the importance of listening and support

One of the priorities in caring for children with kidney disease is to recognize the emotional impact of the disease. Young children, in particular, may have difficulty understanding what is happening to them and expressing their emotions. They may experience feelings of fear, confusion or anger in the face of repetitive treatments and the uncertainty associated with their condition. It is therefore essential to create a climate of **trust**, where the child feels listened to and secure.

Active listening is a key component of emotional support. Children must feel free to express their concerns, pain or frustrations without fear of being judged. Healthcare professionals, especially nurses' aides and pediatric nurses, play a fundamental role in this dialogue, by being available to answer the child's questions and using simple, age-appropriate terms to explain the illness and treatments. For example, instead of using technical terms like "dialysis" or "corticosteroids", it's better to use metaphors that the child can understand, such as "a machine that cleans your blood" or "medicines to help your body feel better".

Another aspect of this support is helping the child to **manage** his **or her emotions**. Dialysis sessions, medical examinations or frequent hospitalizations can be traumatic experiences, and children can feel powerless in the face of what they are going through. **Relaxation techniques**, such as deep breathing or positive visualization, can be taught to children to help them better manage the stress and anxiety associated with care. In addition, **the presence of a psychologist** specialized in pediatrics can be essential, especially for older children or adolescents, who may feel a sense of injustice or isolation as a result of their illness.

Supporting families: essential partners in the care process

The child's parents and family are key players in the day-to-day management of the disease. For them, the shock of learning that their child has severe kidney disease can be devastating. Not only do they have to cope with their own emotions, but they also have to take on the responsibility of looking after their child's well-being, following up on treatments, making sure medical appointments are kept, and monitoring the progress of the disease.

This demands a great deal of **resilience**, and without appropriate support, parents can quickly feel overwhelmed.

It's essential to **provide parents with clear information** about their child's illness, its causes, available treatments, and long-term options. A well-informed parent is one who feels more in control of the situation and can actively participate in care decisions. Doctors and nurses need to take the time to explain the various stages of treatment, answering questions and allaying any concerns. For example, for a child on dialysis, it's important that parents understand not only how the machine works, but also the warning signs to watch out for, such as symptoms of infection or electrolyte imbalance.

In addition to information, **emotional support for parents** is fundamental. Many parents may feel guilty or responsible for their child's illness, even when it is genetic or idiopathic in origin. They may also feel emotionally drained by juggling childcare, work and other family responsibilities. It is therefore crucial to offer them a space to express their emotions, whether through parent **support groups**, where they can exchange experiences and find comfort, or through individual psychological consultations.

The sick child's siblings must not be forgotten. They may feel neglected or jealous of the constant attention their sibling requires. It's important that parents, with the help of healthcare professionals, take the time to explain the situation to all siblings and ensure that each child receives the necessary emotional support.

Adapting to everyday life: reconciling illness and a child's life

Despite the illness, it's important for the child to be able to maintain a normal life as far as possible. This means finding a balance between treatment and age-appropriate activities such as play, school and leisure. Support for sick children must therefore include strategies to help them **reconcile medical care with their needs for socialization and personal development**.

For school-age children, education can become a challenge when they are frequently hospitalized or undergoing heavy treatment. It is essential to put in place appropriate solutions, such as **home schooling** or **hospital school** programs, which enable children to continue their schooling despite medical constraints. These programs are essential not only for their intellectual development, but also for maintaining a social bond with their classmates and preserving a sense of normalcy.

Children should also be encouraged to **take part in activities adapted to their state of health**, such as gentle sports or creative hobbies, in order to preserve their mental and physical well-being. Play is particularly important for younger children, as it enables them to express themselves, temporarily forget about their illness, and boost their self-confidence. Caregivers can integrate playful moments into care, using games or activities to distract the child during medical procedures, for example.

Preparing teenagers for independence: helping them to take charge of their lives

For adolescents with chronic kidney disease, disease management becomes a particular challenge as they approach adulthood. Adolescence is a time of **seeking autonomy** and self-assertion, and adolescents may feel a growing need to take charge of their treatment. This requires specific support to help them **understand their illness**, follow their treatment independently, and take ownership of the medical decisions affecting them.

One of the aims of the support is to enable the teenager to **develop self-management skills**. This includes teaching them how to monitor their health (for example, how to watch their weight or blood pressure), understand the side effects of medication, and manage home dialysis if they are involved. Caregivers can play a key role in providing practical advice and encouraging adolescents to ask questions and actively participate in medical consultations.

However, this autonomy must be accompanied by strong emotional support, as adolescence is also a period marked by **doubts about identity** and questions about the future. Adolescents can feel very frustrated by their illness, which limits their freedom or sets them apart from their peers. Appropriate psychological support can help them overcome these challenges, boost their self-esteem and come to terms with their condition.

- **The psychological impact of treatment on children**: Playful and educational support.

The **provision of playful and educational support** is a central element in the care of children suffering from chronic illnesses, such as those affecting the kidneys. The aim is to create a care environment where children can both learn to better understand their illness and enjoy moments of distraction and relaxation, despite medical constraints. Playful support helps transform often stressful situations into more positive experiences, while the educational approach aims to provide the child with the necessary tools to better apprehend his treatment and develop skills that will help him cope with his illness in a more serene manner. Together, these two dimensions play an essential role in the child's overall well-being.

Play as a tool for support and comfort

Play is an essential part of a child's development, and a natural way for them to interact with the world around them. When illness imposes heavy treatment and hospital stays, play becomes a powerful means of restoring the child's sense of control and normalcy. It creates moments of lightness in an often anxiety-provoking context, helping the child to relax and escape from medical reality.

In a medical context, play can also provide **emotional support**. Sick children, especially those who have to undergo regular or painful treatments such as dialysis or venipunctures, can develop anxiety or fear at the thought of these procedures. Play, as a playful and immersive activity, helps to divert the child's attention during care, reducing stress and perceived pain. For example, the use of interactive video games during dialysis can distract the child from the medical context for a time. In addition, hospital clowns or specialized entertainers play a key role in using play and humor to ease tension.

Play also has a **socializing** function, offering hospitalized children or those undergoing regular treatment the opportunity to bond with other young patients. Sharing moments of play helps children to feel less isolated, to meet other children going through similar situations, and to rediscover a natural, spontaneous space for communication. This is particularly important for children who, because of their illness, are sometimes cut off from school or social life. Group play gives them back a sense of belonging and normalcy.

Teaching approach: learning to understand your illness

The educational approach is another fundamental aspect of support for sick children, especially those suffering from chronic pathologies such as nephrotic syndrome or renal failure. Understanding one's illness and the associated treatments can help children feel more in control, accept the situation better, and become more autonomous in managing their health. However, this understanding needs to be adapted to the child's age, level of development and ability to integrate complex information.

An effective educational approach is based on **simple, appropriate communication**. Caregivers, especially pediatric nurses and health educators, play a crucial role in explaining disease and treatment in an accessible way. For example, for a child with kidney failure, it's important to explain why he or she needs to follow a low-salt or low-potassium diet, and what effects these minerals can have on the body. This can be done through educational games or visual aids, such as illustrated books, videos or interactive drawings.

Educational workshops can also be an effective way of helping children to become involved in their own care. These workshops enable children to learn, in a fun way, how to monitor their health or manage certain aspects of their treatment, such as taking medication or monitoring their diuresis. They can, for example, learn how to use a blood pressure monitor to measure their blood pressure, or how to interpret the results of a urine test. These activities build children's self-confidence and help them better understand the reasons for the care they receive.

For older children, and especially teenagers, the educational approach needs to evolve towards **gradual empowerment**. They can be encouraged to ask questions about their illness, understand the side effects of medication, and actively participate in medical consultations. Their involvement in managing their own health prepares them for the transition to adulthood, when they will be responsible for their own care. Adolescents can, for example, take part in educational programs that introduce them to the basics of self-management, such as scheduling medical appointments or managing treatments at home.

Playful support as a learning lever

Play and educational support are not only intended to entertain or educate children separately: these two dimensions can and should complement each other. Indeed, play can become a powerful **learning tool**. For example, role-playing or dramatization can be used to familiarize children with the medical procedures they are about to undergo. By playing the role of a doctor or nurse, children can better understand what's about to happen to them, and feel less afraid. This playful approach also helps to defuse anxieties linked to the unknown, making care more accessible and less intimidating.

Digital **educational games**, or interactive health apps, are also increasingly used to explain medical concepts in an engaging way. These tools enable children to learn at their own pace, while having fun at the same time. They can, for example, follow interactive courses where they must solve challenges linked to managing their disease, such as eating well to take care of their kidneys or remembering to take their medication. These games reinforce children's understanding and involvement in their treatment, while making learning fun and stimulating.

In addition, play can serve **as** a **channel of expression** for emotions that the child finds difficult to verbalize. Creative activities, such as drawing or painting, can enable children to represent their emotions and fears in ways that are not necessarily verbal. Therapeutic play, supervised by psychologists or educators, can be used to explore the child's feelings about his or her illness, such as anger, sadness or anxiety, and help him or her manage them.

Involving families in playful and educational support

Playful and educational support is not just for caregivers and educators, but also for families, who play a fundamental role in the daily accompaniment of the sick child. Parents and siblings need to be involved in these activities, not only to strengthen the family bond, but also to better understand the challenges the child is going through and help him or her overcome them.

Family workshops, in which parents and children take part in fun and educational activities together, help to strengthen parents' disease management skills. For example, culinary workshops can teach parents and children to cook together dishes adapted to the child's renal diet, while making the experience fun and collaborative. Similarly, educational health games can be used

174

with the family to make everyone aware of the issues involved in treating the child.

Involving the family in these activities also helps **to reduce the isolation** the child may feel. When a child is ill, he may feel different from his siblings or friends, and this difference may be accentuated if care or treatment separates him from the rest of the family. Shared fun and educational activities help to strengthen bonds and create moments of joy and complicity, even in a difficult medical context.

Chapter 14

Palliative care in nephrology

- **End-stage renal disease and the end of life**: Accompanying a patient in nephrology palliative care.

Accompanying a patient in **nephrology palliative care** is a profoundly human process, marked by a holistic approach that takes into account not only physical suffering, but also the psychological, social and spiritual dimensions of the patient's experience. In the context of end-stage chronic kidney disease, palliative care aims to improve the patient's quality of life when curative treatments are no longer effective or appropriate, and to relieve symptoms while respecting the patient's dignity. Nephrology palliative care involves a multidisciplinary approach, attentive listening and a continuous presence with the patient and family.

Understanding the specificities of nephrology palliative care

In the nephrology context, palliative care is often initiated when chronic kidney disease is progressing towards a terminal phase and therapeutic options, such as dialysis or transplantation, are no longer desired or possible. This phase of the disease is marked by a progressive deterioration in renal function, accompanied by complications such as heart failure, electrolyte imbalances, hyperkalemia and profound fatigue. Treatment is no longer focused on curing the disease, but on alleviating **symptoms** and managing the **pain** and **discomfort** associated with them.

The first challenge of palliative care in nephrology is to take into account the **complexity of symptomatology**. Patients may suffer from chronic pain, digestive disorders (such as nausea and vomiting), intense itching (uraemic pruritus), oedema, breathing difficulties and disabling fatigue. Symptom control must be at the heart of support, with particular attention paid to pain management with **appropriate analgesics**, while taking into account renal fragility. Medications must be carefully chosen to avoid aggravating renal failure, which makes pharmacological management more delicate.

A personalized, multidisciplinary approach

Palliative care requires a **multi-disciplinary approach**, involving a variety of healthcare professionals, each contributing their expertise to improve the patient's quality of life. The care team includes nephrologists, specialist nurses, nursing aides, psychologists, dieticians, social workers and, sometimes, spiritual advisors. Each member of the team has a specific role to play, but all work together to ensure that the patient is cared for as a whole.

The nephrologist's role in palliative care is to monitor disease progression, adjust treatments to manage symptoms while avoiding unnecessary interventions, and help the patient and family make informed decisions about end-of-life options. For example, in the advanced stages of renal failure, it may be decided to stop dialysis if it no longer helps to improve quality of life, and to focus care on comfort.

Nurses play a crucial role in the day-to-day care of patients. They are often the first to identify new symptoms or assess the effectiveness of pain relief treatments. Their regular presence at the patient's bedside helps establish a bond of trust, essential for providing emotional support. They ensure that the patient is comfortable, has access to basic care (toileting, hydration, appropriate nutrition), and monitors for signs of distress or worsening general condition.

Palliative care support must be **tailored** to the patient's needs and wishes. This includes not only the relief of physical symptoms, but also consideration of the patient's **personal aspirations and preferences** regarding the end of life. Some patients express specific wishes, such as the desire to remain at home, to limit certain medical interventions, or to receive spiritual support. Respecting these choices is fundamental to ensuring that palliative care is tailored to the individuality of each patient.

Supporting the emotional and psychological dimension

One of the most important aspects of palliative care is **dealing with emotions**. Patients at the end of life often go through phases of **anguish, sadness, anger or resignation** in the face of illness. The announcement of the end of curative treatments can come as a shock, and the patient needs to be accompanied with gentleness and kindness in order to apprehend this new reality. Listening is essential. Caregivers, like loved ones, must know how to be present without imposing, allowing the patient to verbalize his anxieties or regrets, without minimizing his feelings.

Fear of pain and suffering is often one of the main sources of anxiety for patients at the end of life. It is therefore essential to clearly explain to the patient that solutions exist to control pain, and that the care team will do everything possible to ensure his or her comfort. This reassurance helps to ease anxiety and promote a more serene environment.

Psychological support is also essential. Psychologists working in palliative care help patients to cope with illness, express their emotions and manage the anticipated bereavement of their own lives. Some patients also wish to benefit from spiritual support, whether through religious counselors or simply discussions on the meaning of life, death and the aftermath. Respecting the patient's spiritual beliefs and values, without judgment, is an essential component of support.

Supporting families: anticipatory mourning and emotional support

The **families** of nephrology palliative care patients also go through a difficult period, marked by **anticipated bereavement**, anxiety about seeing their loved one suffer, and fear of the unknown. Supporting families is an integral part of palliative care, as their emotional well-being has a direct impact on the patient's quality of life. Relatives need to be helped to understand the disease, the end-of-life stages, and to accept the inevitability of death.

Emotional support for families takes many forms. Caregivers need to be available to answer questions, provide clear and transparent information, and offer a listening space for families to express their fears and grief. Support groups, consultations with psychologists, or even informal discussions with the care team can help lighten the emotional burden families carry.

Caregivers must also ensure that families are not overwhelmed by the **day-to-day care**, especially when the patient is being cared for at home. Caregivers or home help services can be called in to relieve the burden on relatives, enabling them to concentrate on their emotional support role. Relieving the physical and mental burden allows families to spend quality time with their loved ones, which is essential in this phase of life.

Respecting the dignity and wishes of patients at the end of life

One of the fundamental principles of palliative care is **respect for** the patient's **dignity**. It is essential to preserve the patient's autonomy and ability to make end-of-life decisions, wherever possible. This includes respecting the wishes expressed by the patient in **advance directives**, or in discussions with caregivers and family. Patients must be fully informed of their options, and be able to express their preferences regarding treatment, comfort care and the circumstances surrounding their death.

Respect for dignity also involves the way in which the patient is cared for on a daily basis. Maintaining personal hygiene, taking care of appearance, respecting privacy, and ensuring that the patient is comfortable all contribute to this sense of dignity. Even at the end of life, patients must be able to feel valued and respected in their individuality.

- **The importance of quality of life**: relieving symptoms, offering comfort in the final moments.

Relieving symptoms and offering comfort in the last moments of life is at the heart of the palliative approach, where the aim is no longer to cure the disease, but to ensure that the end of life is as serene and peaceful as possible. In this context, care is not limited to the management of physical pain, but also includes comprehensive support aimed at offering the person an optimal **quality of life** despite the progression of the disease. This approach involves not only rigorous symptom control, but also compassionate, caring support that respects the patient's dignity and wishes.

Relieving physical symptoms: a key objective

In palliative care, one of the most crucial aspects is to **relieve the physical symptoms** that can become intense and disabling as the end of life approaches. Patients suffering from advanced chronic illnesses, such as end-stage renal failure, may be confronted with multiple symptoms: **chronic pain, breathing difficulties, nausea, extreme fatigue**, or **digestive disorders**. Each of these symptoms needs to be managed individually, to ensure maximum relief.

Pain management is often a central concern in palliative care. It is essential to ensure that the patient does not suffer unnecessarily. Pain can be relieved with medications ranging from simple analgesics (such as paracetamol) to more potent opioids (such as morphine), depending on the severity and nature of the pain. Dose adjustment must be finely calibrated to offer effective relief without inducing excessive side effects, such as drowsiness or confusion. Caregivers must be attentive to the patient's needs, adjusting treatments as pain progresses, and responding rapidly to any worsening of symptoms.

In addition to pain, patients may suffer **respiratory symptoms** such as shortness of breath (dyspnea), which can be very distressing. Treatments can be put in place to alleviate this sensation of breathlessness, including oxygen therapy, medications to reduce the sensation of breathlessness (such as anxiolytics), and positioning techniques to facilitate breathing. In some cases, simple environmental adjustments, such as opening a window or using a fan, can considerably improve respiratory comfort.

Gastrointestinal symptoms, such as nausea, vomiting or constipation, are also common in terminally ill patients, particularly those on opioid therapy. Caregivers must be alert to these side effects, and implement specific treatments, such as antiemetics for nausea or laxatives to prevent constipation. Every symptom, however minor it may seem, must be taken into account, as it can become a source of considerable suffering if not treated promptly.

Uremic pruritus, common in patients with end-stage renal disease, is intense itching due to the accumulation of toxins in the body. This symptom can be extremely uncomfortable, disrupting sleep and quality of life. Specific treatments, such as soothing creams, antihistamines, or even more frequent dialysis, can be implemented to reduce this symptom.

Providing comfort: attention to the smallest detail

One of the cornerstones of palliative care is to **make** the patient **as comfortable as possible** in their final moments, ensuring that they are physically comfortable and feel emotionally secure. This involves a multitude of small actions and attentions which, when combined, help to create a soothing environment.

Patient positioning is a key factor. A person confined to bed for long periods can quickly develop pain or discomfort due to immobility. Caregivers and nurses must regularly reposition the patient to prevent pressure sores and relieve pressure points. The use of **suitable cushions** and anti-pressure sore mattresses can also help prevent these pains. Sometimes, a simple change of position (such as raising the bed slightly or placing a pillow under the legs) can significantly improve patient comfort.

Personal hygiene is also essential to the patient's well-being. Although some terminally ill people may be too weak to wash themselves, caregivers can offer them appropriate grooming, which is not only important for physical comfort but also for preserving the patient's dignity. The use of moist towelettes, mild products and care for appearance (such as brushing hair or moisturizing skin) can provide a feeling of freshness and well-being, even as health deteriorates.

Hydration and nutrition must also be adapted to the patient's condition. When appetite diminishes or swallowing becomes difficult, it is essential to respect the patient's needs without forcing him or her to eat or drink. Solutions may include small, easy-to-swallow bites, thickened liquids, or even artificial nutrition if the patient and family so wish. The important thing is to respect the patient's limits, avoiding any additional discomfort.

Emotional comfort: offering a caring presence

Emotional comfort is as important as physical comfort, and is often what determines whether the last moments of life are lived in serenity. The end of life can be a time of great **anxiety** for the patient, who often feels vulnerable and confronted with deep-seated fears, such as that of pain, suffering or death itself. A **constant**, caring **human presence** is essential to allay these fears.

One of the most important aspects of support is **active listening**. It's about being present for the patient, listening without judging, without trying to minimize their anxieties, and offering them a space where they can express their fears, regrets or wishes. Often, it's not necessary to have ready-made answers. Simply being there, holding the patient's hand or offering a reassuring word, is enough to create a climate of emotional security. This caring presence is just as important for loved ones, who may also feel helpless in the face of a loved one's imminent death.

Some people find comfort in **spirituality** or **religion**, and it is essential to respect patients' beliefs and allow them to live out their final moments in accordance with their convictions. This can take the form of the presence of a spiritual advisor, the practice of religious rituals, or simply discussions about the meaning of life and death. It is important that caregivers adopt an open, non-directive approach, letting patients choose how they wish to live out these moments.

Supporting loved ones: an essential part of the final moments

In addition to patient care, **palliative care** also includes **family support**. For loved ones, the last moments of life can be particularly trying. They are confronted with the pain of losing a loved one, the fear of seeing them suffer, and often a sense of helplessness. The role of caregivers is not only to accompany the patient, but also to **support families**, helping them to understand the different stages of end-of-life, informing them about what they can expect, and offering them a space to express their emotions.

It's important to involve loved ones in care, if they so wish. They can be invited to take part in simple gestures, such as holding the patient's hand, talking to him, or helping him to settle down. These shared moments help maintain a strong **emotional bond** and give meaning to the final moments. Caregivers must also offer psychological support to families, listening to their fears and questions, and helping them to come to terms with their loved one's end of life.

- **Bereavement support for loved ones**: how to help families through this delicate phase.

Supporting families during the delicate phase of a loved one's palliative care is an essential component of end-of-life care. Families, like patients, are going through a period of profound emotional and psychological upheaval. They face the pain of impending loss, the uncertainty of disease progression, and the weight of care decisions. This support must be practical, emotional and psychological, while respecting the individual needs of family members, who may react differently to the situation.

Offer a sympathetic and caring ear

Supporting families starts with **active, sympathetic listening**. Faced with the suffering of a loved one, families often feel a complex mix of emotions: sadness, fear, frustration, sometimes even anger or guilt. It is vital to create a space where they can **freely express** these feelings without fear of being judged. Caregivers, especially nurses, orderlies, psychologists and doctors, need to be available to answer questions, listen to concerns, and offer clear, reassuring explanations of the patient's condition and the course of care.

This listening must be marked by **empathy**, recognizing that each family member may experience the anticipated mourning process in a unique way. Some may want to talk at length about their emotions, while others may remain withdrawn or need moments of silence. The role of caregivers is to **adapt to each situation**, without forcing people to talk, but remaining present and open at all times when the need for communication arises.

Providing clear, appropriate information

One of the greatest stresses for families in this delicate phase is the **uncertainty** surrounding the evolution of the patient's state of health. Families may feel lost or helpless in the face of symptoms, treatments and the progressive deterioration of their loved one.

That's why it's essential to **provide clear**, understandable **information** adapted to their level of medical knowledge. Caregivers need to explain, in simple words, what the family can expect in the coming days or weeks, describing the signs of disease progression, the care options available, and the means put in place to ensure the patient's comfort.

This transparency helps **reduce** families' **anxiety** by enabling them to better anticipate the steps ahead. For example, explaining why certain medications are administered, how pain is managed, or what certain physical signs mean (such as changes in breathing or increased sleepiness) helps families prepare emotionally and avoid misinterpretations or anxiety.

Helping with decision-making: support for difficult choices

Families are often faced with **difficult decisions** at the end of life, particularly when it comes to choosing between continuing certain treatments or concentrating solely on comfort care. These choices can be a source of anguish and guilt, as loved ones may feel they are "betraying" the patient by stopping an active treatment, or may fear making a decision they don't fully understand.

The role of caregivers is to **guide families** through these choices, explaining with compassion and clarity the different options available, their implications, and the expected outcomes. Families need to be reassured that choosing palliative care or limiting medical interventions does not mean "giving up", but rather respecting the patient's wishes and maximizing their comfort. By taking the time to discuss the patient's **advance directives**, where they exist, and encouraging open dialogue within the family, caregivers help to lighten the burden of decision-making.

Encouraging participation in care and sharing moments

Taking an active part in the care of a loved one at the end of life can be a way for families to stay **involved** and maintain a strong bond with the patient. Some family members may find comfort in getting involved in everyday gestures, such as helping to give a glass of water, holding hands, or simply being present during moments of care. Caregivers can encourage this involvement, while ensuring that it does not become too much of a burden for the family. It is important to offer them moments of **respite** when necessary, reminding them that they are not alone in bearing this responsibility.

What's more, creating **moments of sharing** between patient and family is crucial. These can be simple moments, such as reading a book, listening to music together, looking at photos, or simply being present in silence. These moments help strengthen the emotional bond and let families create meaningful memories with their loved ones, even in this terminal phase. The support of caregivers, who ensure that these moments take place in optimal conditions (for example, by making sure that the patient is comfortable and that pain is well controlled), is essential.

Offering psychological support: accompanying anticipated bereavement

Anticipatory grief is a reality for families whose loved one is at the end of life. They begin to cope with the loss even before the death occurs, which can generate a complex mix of emotions, from sadness and anger to guilt and sometimes relief as the patient's suffering comes to an end. **Psychological support** is essential to help families navigate through these emotions and find ways to express and understand them.

Psychologists and palliative care counsellors can offer **individual or family interviews** to help verbalize emotions, anticipate bereavement, and find ways to support the patient while taking care of their own well-being. Support groups, where families can meet others in a similar situation, also provide a space for sharing and mutual understanding, helping to break the isolation that some loved ones may feel.

Ensuring continuity of support after death

Family support doesn't end with the patient's death. The period following the loss can be particularly difficult, and families may feel a deep need to be **accompanied in their grief**. Palliative care teams can stay in touch with loved ones, offer bereavement resources (such as consultations with psychologists, discussion groups or grief counsellors), and direct them to **appropriate support services**.

It's important to recognize that each family member may experience bereavement differently, with some feeling profound sadness, others relief, and sometimes a mixture of both. Caregivers must be careful not to minimize these reactions, and to offer a space where each emotion is welcomed with respect and kindness.

Chapter 15

Environment and risk management in the nephrology department

- **Hygiene and infection prevention in nephrology**: Specific precautions for dialysis and immunocompromised patients.

Patients undergoing dialysis or immunodepression are **particularly vulnerable**, due to their fragile state of health and the treatments they receive. For these patients, specific precautions must be put in place to prevent infections, minimize complications related to medical care, and ensure a safe care environment. Risks are heightened for both these categories of patients, due to the suppression or alteration of their immune defenses, or the need for regular invasive procedures such as dialysis. Understanding and applying these precautions can help reduce the risk of serious complications, and better protect these vulnerable patients.

Infection prevention: a central issue

Dialysis and **immunocompromised** patients are at increased risk of infections, whether bacterial, viral or fungal in origin. Dialysis patients, particularly those with arteriovenous fistulas or central catheters, are at risk of infection from vascular access devices. Similarly, immunocompromised patients, whether due to immunosuppressive therapy (as after transplantation) or autoimmune disease, have a reduced ability to fight pathogens, exposing them to serious and often difficult-to-treat infections.

Strict hygiene of hands and medical equipment

The first line of defense against infection is **rigorous hand hygiene**, for healthcare professionals, patients and their families. Washing hands with soap and water, or using a hydroalcoholic solution before and after each contact with the patient or medical equipment, is essential to prevent the transmission of germs. This is all the more important during dialysis sessions, where the risk of infection is high due to regular handling of the fistula or catheter.

As far as **medical equipment** is concerned, each device must be carefully disinfected or sterilized before being used on an immunocompromised or dialyzed patient. Care teams must follow strict disinfection protocols to avoid cross-contamination. In the case of dialysis catheters or venous lines, **aseptic handling techniques** are essential to prevent infection of the insertion site, which can develop into serious infections such as septicemia.

Vaccinations and prophylaxis

Patients who are immunocompromised or on dialysis should benefit from **enhanced vaccination protection**, as they are more susceptible to serious infections such as influenza, pneumococcal disease and hepatitis B. Vaccination against influenza is recommended every year, as is the pneumococcal vaccine, which protects against potentially fatal respiratory infections. In addition, vaccination against hepatitis B is particularly important for dialysis patients, as they may be exposed to contamination risks during treatment.

In addition to vaccines, **prophylactic measures** can be put in place, notably to prevent fungal or bacterial infections in patients undergoing immunosuppressive treatment after transplantation. These preventive treatments, such as antibiotics or antifungals, reduce the risk of infection at a time when immune defenses are severely weakened.

Extra precautions during epidemics

During **epidemic** periods, such as that of influenza or COVID-19, immunocompromised or dialysis patients need even greater protection. This includes limiting visits, systematically using **personal protective equipment** (such as masks), and isolating patients showing symptoms of infection. Dialysis centers must implement **strict triage protocols** to identify patients at risk of infection and adapt their management, for example by dialyzing them in separate rooms or at the end of the day to avoid contact with other patients.

Special care for dialysis patients

Dialysis patients, whether on hemodialysis or peritoneal dialysis, require special care to minimize the risk of treatment-related complications. Hemodialysis, in particular, exposes patients to frequent manipulation of their vascular system, requiring extra vigilance.

Preventing vascular access site infections

One of the most serious complications for **hemodialysis** patients is **infection of the vascular access site**, whether an arteriovenous fistula or a central catheter. Caregivers must follow rigorous disinfection procedures before each puncture. This includes careful cleaning of the skin around the insertion site and the use of antiseptic solutions to avoid bacterial contamination. In addition, it's important to regularly monitor the access site for any signs of infection, such as redness, swelling, warmth or discharge. If infection is suspected, prompt treatment with antibiotics may be necessary to prevent the infection spreading and becoming systemic.

Arteriovenous fistula monitoring

The **arteriovenous fistula** is the preferred access route for dialysis, as it presents less risk of infection than catheters. However, it can also be prone to complications, such as **thrombosis** (clot formation) or stenosis (narrowing of the vessels). It is therefore essential that caregivers and patients regularly monitor the **fistula murmur** (the sound or vibration that indicates good blood flow) and report any changes in its appearance or functionality. Prompt intervention can help prevent more serious complications, such as fistula loss.

Water and nutritional balance

Dialysis patients must follow **strict diets** to maintain adequate fluid and electrolyte balance. Particular attention must be paid to fluid, sodium, potassium and phosphorus intake, as inadequate management can lead to serious complications, such as hyperkalemia, pulmonary edema or cardiac disorders. Caregivers, in collaboration with dieticians, must regularly assess patients' **dietary intake** and adjust dietary recommendations according to the results of biological analyses and the patient's clinical evolution.

Special care for immunocompromised patients

Immunocompromised patients, whether due to immunosuppressive treatments (after kidney transplantation or due to autoimmune diseases) or to an underlying medical condition, require specific care to **reduce the risk of infections** and monitor for early signs of complications.

Post-renal transplant follow-up

Kidney transplant patients are treated with immunosuppressive drugs to prevent graft rejection. Although these drugs are essential, they weaken the patient's immune defenses, considerably increasing the risk of infections. It is therefore crucial to maintain **regular medical follow-up**, including frequent blood tests to monitor kidney function and detect any signs of rejection, infection or drug toxicity.

Regular consultations also ensure that the patient is following recommendations concerning hygiene measures, medication intake and dietary restrictions. In the event of fever, respiratory or digestive symptoms, immunocompromised patients should consult their doctor immediately, as an infection can quickly become serious.

Avoiding sources of infection

For immunocompromised patients, it's essential to **limit exposure to potential sources of infection**. This includes contact with sick people, crowded places, or environments likely to contain germs, such as hospitals or clinics. At home, relatives and caregivers should take **extra precautions**, such as wearing masks in case of colds or flu, regularly disinfecting surfaces, and avoiding bringing sick people near the patient.

Patients should also avoid certain **high-risk foods**, such as unpasteurized products, raw meat or fish, and poorly washed vegetables, which can be carriers of serious foodborne infections. Caregivers and dieticians can provide **tailored nutritional advice** to ensure that the patient's diet is both safe and balanced.

- **Medical waste management**: sorting protocol and infectious risk management.

Triage protocols and **infectious risk management** are crucial elements in ensuring patient safety, particularly in settings where vulnerability to infection is high, such as dialysis patients, immunocompromised patients or those suffering from chronic diseases. These protocols are designed to prevent the spread of infections within care facilities, and to rapidly identify patients at risk, so as to offer them appropriate care while limiting the risk of cross-contamination. Rigorous implementation of these protocols is essential to protect both patients and caregivers, and to guarantee a safe care environment.

Triage protocol: identify and isolate at-risk patients

Screening patients as soon as they enter a healthcare facility is a crucial step in preventing the spread of infection, particularly in epidemic situations or when contagious diseases are present.

Triage consists of **rapidly assessing** the health status of patients as soon as they are admitted, in order to detect those who show signs of infection or who are likely to spread an infectious disease. This process is particularly important in departments with fragile patients, such as nephrology or oncology, where the risk of infection can have serious consequences.

Early detection of signs of infection

When screening, it's essential to look out for **early signs** of infection, such as fever, cough, breathing difficulties, or digestive symptoms such as diarrhea. A **systematic questionnaire** is often used to gather information on the patient's symptoms, recent medical history, and any contact with sick people. This assessment enables patients to be **categorized** according to their level of infectious risk, so that their care can be adapted immediately.

Rapid triage is all the more important in departments such as dialysis centers, where many immunocompromised patients are regularly present. A patient showing signs of infection, whether from a respiratory illness such as influenza or a bacterial infection, must be **isolated** immediately to avoid contamination of other patients. It is often necessary to set up a dedicated area or cubicle for the care of infected patients, to ensure physical separation from other patients.

Isolation of high-risk patients

If a patient is identified as a potential carrier of a contagious infection, appropriate **isolation** must be implemented. This can be done in special rooms or individual cubicles equipped with ventilation systems to prevent the spread of airborne germs. It is also possible to implement **isolation at home**, in cases where this is recommended, with clear instructions given to patients and their families on the precautions to be taken to avoid contamination of those around them.

Caregivers caring for patients at high risk of infection must wear **personal protective equipment (PPE)**, such as masks, gloves, gowns and protective glasses. Appropriate use of PPE is crucial to prevent caregivers themselves from becoming vectors of transmission. Strict protocols for **donning and doffing** PPE must be followed, with systematic disinfection after every contact with a patient at risk.

Infectious risk management: a systematic, preventive approach

Infectious risk management is based on a series of **preventive** and **curative measures** designed to limit the transmission of pathogens within healthcare establishments. These measures are adapted to the different types of infection (bacterial, viral, fungal) and are implemented according to the risk level of the patient and his or her environment. Infectious risk management is a process that involves not only nursing staff, but also patients, visitors and families.

Hand and surface hygiene: an absolute priority

Hand hygiene is one of the pillars of infection prevention. Caregivers, patients and visitors must be trained in the importance of washing their hands before and after each contact with the patient or potentially contaminated surfaces. The use of **hydroalcoholic solutions** is widespread in healthcare establishments, and should be systematized in areas where the risk of infection is high, such as dialysis or oncology departments.

Frequently touched **surfaces**, such as door handles, beds, medical devices or care carts, need to be regularly **disinfected**. Cleaning protocols include the use of disinfectants effective against common pathogens, such as resistant bacteria (e.g. methicillin-resistant Staphylococcus aureus) or viruses (e.g. SARS-CoV-2).

Specially trained cleaning teams should be in charge of regular maintenance in high-risk areas.

Controlling nosocomial infections

Nosocomial infections, i.e. infections contracted in hospital, represent a major risk, particularly for immunocompromised patients or those on dialysis. These infections can occur during invasive procedures (catheterization, surgery, dialysis) or as a result of the hospital environment. Infectious risk management in this context relies on rigorous **sterilization protocols** for all equipment used (needles, catheters, medical devices) and particular attention to **asepsis** during care. Caregivers must be trained in best practices to reduce the risk of cross-contamination, notably by using single-use equipment or sterilizing between uses.

Dialysis **catheters**, for example, are frequent entry points for infections. A strict catheter management protocol, including handling with sterile techniques and regular monitoring, helps reduce the risk of vascular access-related infections. It is also essential to monitor access sites for **signs of infection**, such as redness, swelling, warmth or pain, so that prompt action can be taken if infection is suspected.

Patient and staff flow management

In high-risk environments, such as dialysis centers or intensive care units, **managing the flow of patients** and staff is an important component of infection prevention. Patients who are immunocompromised or on dialysis must be protected from contact with infected patients. This may involve setting up specific circuits to avoid cross-fertilization, organizing care for these patients at dedicated times, or reserving specific treatment rooms for them.

Caregivers handling these patients need to be **deployed accordingly**, ensuring that they do not move from a patient at risk of infection to a vulnerable patient without following strict hygiene protocols. Facilities can set up **buffer zones**, where staff wash their hands, change clothes or use PPE before entering at-risk units.

Epidemiological surveillance and continuing education

A key element of infectious risk management is **epidemiological surveillance**, which enables the early detection of any signs of an epidemic or an increase in the number of cases of infection in a facility. Care teams must be trained to report **suspected** or confirmed **cases of** infection, whether nosocomial or community-acquired. Protocols for **notifying** health authorities make it possible to monitor the evolution of infections and adjust preventive measures accordingly.

In addition, **ongoing training** of nursing staff is essential to ensure proper management of infectious risks. Caregivers must be regularly trained in new protocols for disinfection, sterilization, isolation, and management of infected patients. Regular audits can be carried out to ensure that good practices are being followed, and to identify areas for improvement.

- **Staff and patient safety**: Prevent risks associated with patient movements and transfers.

Preventing the risks associated with **patient movements and transfers** is a major challenge in healthcare, both for patient and caregiver safety. Patients, especially those with chronic illnesses, the elderly or bedridden, are particularly vulnerable to accidents during transfers, whether they involve movement in bed, transferring from bed to a chair, or assisting with walking. A poor transfer can result in falls, fractures or muscular injuries, while for caregivers, poor posture when moving or lifting a patient can lead to musculoskeletal disorders. Implementing **appropriate transfer protocols** and using safe techniques can help prevent these risks and ensure a safer care environment for all.

Assessment of the patient's motor skills

Before proceeding with any movement or transfer, it is essential to accurately assess the patient's **motor skills**. Every patient has different levels of mobility and strength, and this assessment helps determine the type of assistance required and the degree of autonomy the patient can retain. This assessment takes several factors into account:

- **Muscular strength**: Can he stand up on his own? Does he have enough strength in his lower limbs to support his weight when standing?
- **Balance**: Can he stand upright without tipping over? Can he maintain his balance when sitting down or moving around?
- **Coordination**: Is he able to coordinate his movements to walk or turn?
- **Pain**: Does he suffer from pain that could limit his movements or make a transfer more difficult?

Once this assessment has been carried out, the caregiver can determine whether the patient can actively participate in the transfer, or whether full assistance is required. For example, a patient with generalized weakness or significant loss of balance will often require the use of **technical aids** for transfers, such as a patient lift or transfer belt.

Use of technical aids to secure transfers

Technical aids are essential for safe patient transfers and movements. They help limit the risk of falls and protect caregivers from injuries caused by overexertion or inappropriate postures. Among these aids, several are commonly used, depending on patients' specific needs:

- **Patient lift**: This is one of the most widely used pieces of equipment for patients who are totally dependent or unable to move about on their own. Patient lifts enable a person to be lifted safely from a bed to a chair, or vice versa, while limiting physical effort for caregivers. Both fixed and mobile lifts are available, for use directly at the patient's bedside or in other parts of the facility.

- **Transfer belts**: For patients able to participate partially in their transfer, transfer belts provide secure support. They enable caregivers to hold the patient by the waist or hips during a sit-to-stand transfer or short trip. They reinforce the patient's stability while providing a secure support point for caregivers.

- **Walkers or canes**: These devices enable patients with walking difficulties to move around more independently, while reducing the risk of falls. The choice between a walker, a tripod cane or a classic cane depends on the degree of support required by the patient.

- **Transfer board**: Used for patients who are unable to stand, the transfer board enables a patient to be moved from bed to wheelchair or other support without having to be lifted entirely. This device is particularly useful for patients whose mobility is very limited, but who need to be moved frequently.

The use of these technical aids must be accompanied by **appropriate training** for caregivers. Improper handling of this equipment can lead to accidents, so it is essential that medical staff are trained in good practice and appropriate lifting techniques.

Manual transfer techniques and adapted postures

For patients able to participate partially in their transfer, or when the use of a patient lift is not necessary, caregivers need to know and apply safe **manual transfer techniques**. These techniques are based on the principles of **biomechanics** and **adapted postures**, designed to reduce the physical effort required of caregivers while ensuring a smooth, safe transfer for the patient.

- **Center of gravity principle**: During manual transfers, caregivers should keep their center of gravity low and close to the patient. This minimizes the strain on back and lower limb muscles, reducing the risk of injury. Using the legs to lift or guide the patient is recommended, rather than straining the back.

- **Foot positioning**: The caregiver should adopt a **stable posture**, with feet hip-width apart, to distribute weight and ensure stability. Transferring is done by bending the knees, keeping the back straight and using leg strength to lift or support the patient. This posture helps avoid twisting of the back, a frequent cause of injury among caregivers.

- **Synchronized lifting**: When several caregivers are involved in a transfer, it's essential to **coordinate movements**. Counting out loud before lifting or moving a patient ensures that everyone acts at the same time, guaranteeing a smoother transfer and reducing the risk of accidents.

- **Encourage patient participation**: Even partially dependent patients can often contribute to the transfer, making the process easier and more autonomous. Caregivers should clearly explain each step of the transfer to the patient, and encourage them to use their arms, legs or trunk to support the movement. This can also help boost the patient's confidence in his or her physical abilities.

Falls prevention: making walking safer

Falls are one of the main risks associated with patient transfers and movements, particularly for the elderly or patients suffering from muscular weakness or balance disorders. To prevent these accidents, a number of measures need to be implemented at different levels:

- **Environmental layout**: It's essential to ensure that the space around the patient is clear and safe. Obstacles such as carpets, electrical cables or bulky furniture must be removed, and lighting must be sufficient to prevent the patient tripping or slipping. In bathrooms, **grab bars** and non-slip mats can be installed to make moving around safer.

- **Suitable footwear**: Patients must wear **suitable shoes or slippers** with a good grip on the ground to avoid slipping. Open-toed shoes or slippery stockings are to be avoided, as they considerably increase the risk of falling.

- **Walking aids**: Patients with reduced mobility need to be equipped with **walking aids** (such as canes or walkers) to help them get around. These devices provide additional stability and reduce pressure on weakened joints and muscles.

- **Monitoring and assistance**: Caregivers must always be **present and attentive** when moving or transferring patients at risk. They must remain close to the patient, ready to intervene in the event of imminent imbalance or fall. In some cases, it may be necessary to provide continuous assistance for very frail patients, especially when moving over short distances.

Ongoing training for caregivers: guaranteeing safety

Ongoing training for caregivers is essential to prevent risks associated with patient movements and transfers. This training must include both theoretical knowledge of biomechanics and safety principles, and regular practical exercises to help caregivers master transfer techniques and the use of technical aids.

Healthcare facilities must also implement **regular audits** to assess the quality of transfer practices and detect any breaches of safety protocols. Simulation workshops or specific training courses can be organized for caregivers, so that they can perfect their skills and work in a synchronized team.

Conclusion

The caregiver, a pillar of modern nephrology

- **The heart of the profession: care, humanity and technicality**: combining the science of care and human accompaniment.

The nursing profession is deeply rooted in a duality that blends the **science of care** with **human accompaniment**. Both a health technician and a guardian of humanity, the caregiver must combine these two dimensions to offer comprehensive care, which is not limited to clinical management, but also encompasses listening, compassion and understanding of patients' emotional needs. This dual role is demonstrated every day in professional practice, where the technical nature of care is accompanied by constant attention to the individual, his or her experience and dignity.

The scientific aspect: technical expertise at the service of care

The **heart of care** lies in solid technical skills and a mastery of medical science. In an increasingly complex and technologically advanced healthcare environment, caregivers must possess in-depth knowledge of medical pathologies, treatments and procedures. The science of care involves knowing how to use and interpret cutting-edge medical technologies, ensuring rapid and precise interventions, and adjusting care according to the patient's evolving condition.

For example, in the care of dialysis patients, the use of devices such as dialysis machines or the monitoring of vascular access requires a high degree of technical expertise. Caregivers need to master these tools perfectly to guarantee patient safety, prevent complications and ensure treatment efficacy. This includes continuous monitoring of **vital signs**, adjustment of dialysis parameters, management of sophisticated medical equipment, and interpretation of test results. Every technical gesture must be precise, measured and based on a thorough scientific understanding of the human body and the pathologies being treated.

The role of caregivers is not limited to the application of technical gestures; they must also understand and follow rigorous **medical protocols**, while keeping abreast of therapeutic advances. The constant evolution of treatments, best practice recommendations and medical technologies requires healthcare professionals to keep up to date with the latest developments. Their technical expertise is a guarantee of safety for the patient, who can count on high-quality care tailored to his or her needs and in line with current medical standards.

Human support: constant listening and empathy

However, care cannot be reduced to a mere technical dimension. Technicality, while essential, must always be accompanied by a **human dimension** based on empathy, listening and consideration for the whole person. The caregiver is at the heart of the patient-caregiver relationship, and it is this relationship, founded on trust, that enables us to give meaning to technical acts and make the experience of care more bearable for the patient.

Human support involves **active listening**, where the caregiver is attentive to the patient's concerns, anxieties and expectations. This means taking into account not only the physical symptoms, but also the **emotions** that accompany the illness. A patient faced with a serious pathology, such as kidney failure or cancer, often goes through periods of doubt, fear and even depression. The caregiver, by being present, listening without judging and offering words of comfort, plays a vital role in helping the patient overcome these difficult moments.

Empathy is one of the essential qualities of a caregiver. It enables us to put ourselves in the patient's shoes, to understand how they feel, and to adapt care to their emotional state. For example, an anxious patient prior to surgery or a dialysis session will benefit not only from technical explanations of how the treatment is to be carried out, but also from emotional support to allay his or her fears. This may involve simple gestures such as holding the patient's hand, answering questions in a reassuring manner, or explaining each stage of the treatment to reduce the feeling of loss of control.

This human accompaniment is not limited to the patient, but often extends to his or her **family**, who are also going through a period of uncertainty and stress. The caregiver then becomes a key contact for relatives, explaining the medical situation clearly, answering their questions and reassuring them about the quality of the care provided. The ability to manage families' emotions, while maintaining a professional approach, is a fundamental aspect of the caregiver's role.

Combining technical expertise and humanity: an integrated approach to care

One of the great strengths of the nursing profession lies in its ability to **combine** the technical aspect of care with human accompaniment. Technical skills and empathy are not in opposition, but complement each other to offer comprehensive care, where the patient's body and mind are considered inseparably. It is in this combination that the essence of care lies, where every technical gesture is accompanied by special attention to the individual.

Palliative care is a perfect illustration of this **dual dimension**. In this end-of-life approach, the primary goal is no longer healing, but comfort and quality of life. Technical care, such as pain management, symptom monitoring or treatment adjustment, is essential to relieve physical suffering. But it is also the human aspects of care - presence, listening, accompanying in the final moments - that make all the difference. Here, the caregiver becomes a **guide**, capable of maintaining a subtle balance between medical interventions and respect for the patient's emotional and spiritual needs.

Another example is the **care of chronic patients**, such as those suffering from kidney failure requiring regular dialysis. Technical care is undeniable: machines must be mastered, vitals monitored and treatment parameters adjusted. But these patients, often exhausted by years of treatment, also need constant emotional support. The caregiver, by providing technical care while maintaining a relationship of trust and support with the patient, becomes a key player in maintaining their overall well-being.

The ethical dimension: respecting patient dignity and autonomy

Finally, combining technical expertise and humanity also means taking into account the **ethical dimension** of care. Every patient is a unique individual, with his or her own values, beliefs and preferences. Caregivers must always ensure that these aspects are respected, even in complex medical situations. This means not only providing quality care, but also **respecting** patients' **dignity**, giving them the information they need to participate in decisions concerning their health, and respecting their choices, even when they differ from medical recommendations.

Respect for patient **autonomy** is another fundamental aspect of this ethic. Patients must be given transparent information about their state of health and treatment options, so that they can make informed decisions about their care. This transparency, together with a relationship of trust with the caregiver, enables patients to feel fully involved in their care, which is essential to maintaining their dignity and well-being, even in the face of serious illness.

- **The future of nephrology care**: Evolving practices and new technologies on the horizon.

The **future of nephrology care** looks bright, marked by evolving medical practices and the integration of new technologies that are gradually transforming the way kidney disease is diagnosed, treated and monitored. These advances aim to improve patients' quality of life, offer more personalized treatments and push back the boundaries of current care. Nephrology, already a highly technical discipline with treatments such as dialysis and kidney transplantation, is preparing for a future in which care will be more connected, more efficient and, above all, more patient-centered.

Towards more preventive and personalized nephrology

One of the major developments on the horizon is the shift towards **more preventive medicine**, where the aim is no longer simply to treat advanced kidney disease, but to **prevent its onset or progression**. This approach is made possible by advances in the early detection of kidney disease, notably through the use of **biomarkers** and increasingly sophisticated imaging techniques. These tools make it possible to identify signs of kidney damage even before clinical symptoms appear, paving the way for earlier and potentially more effective treatments.

The nephrology of tomorrow will also be marked by **personalized medicine**, where treatments will be tailored to individual patient characteristics. Genomic analysis and **precision medicine** technologies **will play** a central role in this evolution. By identifying specific genetic profiles, it will be possible to determine which patients are most at risk of developing certain kidney diseases, such as polycystic kidney disease, or to assess individual response to treatments. In this way, nephrologists will be able to tailor care to the patient's genetic profile, limiting side effects and maximizing treatment efficacy.

Artificial intelligence (AI) tools are also beginning to transform nephrology. AI can analyze huge amounts of data from medical records, lab results and imaging, to predict the progression of kidney disease or detect early complications. Algorithms can provide treatment recommendations or help nephrologists adjust drug doses according to subtle changes in the patient's state of health. These advances will enable **treatments to be personalized** in a much more refined and dynamic way, taking into account the constant evolution of kidney disease.

Connected dialysis and wearable technologies

Dialysis, currently one of the most burdensome treatments for kidney failure patients, is undergoing a revolution thanks to technological advances. The future of dialysis is moving towards treatments that are more **autonomous, portable** and, above all, better adapted to patients' lifestyles.

Portable dialysis machines, which are still in the development phase, promise to free patients from the constraints of in-center dialysis sessions. These devices enable daily dialysis to be carried out at home or even on the move, offering increased **flexibility** and greater comfort. The aim is to make dialysis less invasive and more suited to patients' daily lives, enabling them to continue working, traveling or taking part in social activities without being restricted by the rigid schedules of in-center dialysis sessions. These portable machines use innovative technologies to reduce the volume of fluid needed for dialysis and make the process less cumbersome.

Another promising development is **connected hemodialysis**. Thanks to sensors integrated into dialysis machines and wearable devices, caregivers can monitor vital parameters and the quality of a patient's dialysis remotely, in real time. These data are transmitted via digital platforms to nephrologists and specialized nurses, who can adjust treatment parameters to suit the patient's condition without the need to travel. This type of remote monitoring enables **faster reaction** in the event of complications and better adaptation of treatment to the patient's daily needs.

At the same time, **automated home dialysis** (such as automated peritoneal dialysis) is becoming increasingly popular. New technologies are simplifying processes and making nocturnal dialysis more accessible, enabling patients to be treated while they sleep, without interrupting their daily routine. What's more, intelligent systems can monitor the quality of dialysis during the night and automatically alert caregivers in the event of a problem, improving the safety and efficiency of treatment.

Bioengineering and artificial organs: a promising future for kidney transplantation

Today, **kidney** transplantation remains one of the best treatment options for patients with end-stage renal failure, but organ shortages and complications associated with immunosuppressive treatments pose major challenges. However, research into **bioengineering** and **artificial organs** is opening up fascinating prospects for the future.

One of the most promising advances is the development of **artificial bioreins**, implantable devices that could replace the functions of damaged kidneys without the need for immunosuppressive treatments. These bioreins, still in the experimental phase, combine filtration technologies and artificial kidney cells to reproduce the kidney's functions of toxin filtration, electrolyte regulation and water balance. This innovation could revolutionize the management of kidney failure, offering an alternative to transplantation and dialysis, while limiting side effects.

At the same time, advances in **3D tissue printing** suggest the possibility of creating **bioartificial organs**, such as kidneys, from a patient's own cells. This would eliminate the risk of organ rejection and dependence on immunosuppressive treatments, while addressing the chronic shortage of kidneys available for transplantation. 3D printing makes it possible to recreate complex kidney structures, with functional cells capable of filtering blood and regulating metabolic waste, although this technology is still in its infancy.

The impact of connected technologies and telemedicine

Telemedicine and **connected technologies** will play a central role in the future of nephrology care. With the number of patients suffering from chronic diseases on the rise, and the need for regular follow-up, connected health technologies will help **relieve overcrowding in care centers**, while ensuring continuous, personalized monitoring.

Mobile applications for monitoring vitals, such as blood pressure, weight or electrolyte levels, enable patients to track their health status in real time and share this data directly with their medical team. This enables more proactive management of renal failure and early detection of complications. These tools also foster greater **autonomy for patients**, by actively involving them in the management of their own health. In the event of an imbalance in vitals, caregivers can be alerted automatically and intervene before the situation deteriorates.

Telemedicine enables nephrologists to carry out consultations at a distance, which is particularly useful for patients living in rural areas or for those who have difficulty travelling. Videoconference consultations, combined with data transmitted by connected devices, offer both responsive and personalized follow-up, while reducing the need for frequent travel for routine appointments. This approach is becoming essential as we seek to maximize resources while improving the quality of care.

The emergence of biotherapies and regenerative treatments

Another fast-growing field is that of **biotherapies** and **regenerative treatments**. **Stem cells** and gene therapy offer unprecedented prospects for treating kidney disease. The idea of being able to regenerate damaged kidney tissue using stem cells opens the way to treatments that could **repair the kidneys**, rather than simply compensate for their failure.

Gene therapies, meanwhile, are being explored to correct the genetic abnormalities responsible for certain inherited kidney diseases, such as polycystic kidney disease. These therapies could make it possible to intervene at an early stage of the disease, slowing or preventing its progression before the kidneys are seriously damaged.

www.ingramcontent.com/pod-product-compliance
Lightning Source LLC
Chambersburg PA
CBHW072151290526
45794CB00004B/1476